Current Clinical Strategies

Medicine

2002-2003 Edition

Paul D. Chan, MD
Executive Editor

Michael Safani, PharmD
Assistant Clinical Professor
School of Pharmacy
University of California, San Francisco

Peter J. Winkle, MD
Associate Editor

Current Clinical Strategies Publishing

www.ccspublishing.com/ccs

Digital Book for Palm, Pocket PC, Windows and Macintosh

Purchasers of this book may download the digital book and updates for Palm, Pocket PC, Windows and Macintosh. The digital books can be downloaded at the Current Clinical Strategies Publishing Internet site:

www.ccspublishing.com/ccs

Current Clinical Strategies Publishing
27071 Cabot Road
Laguna Hills, California 92653-7012
Phone: 800-331-8227 or 949-348-8404
Fax: 800-965-9420 or 949-348-8405
E-mail: info@ccspublishing.com
Internet: www.ccspublishing.com/ccs

Printed in USA   ISBN 1929622-20-1

Contents

Medical Documentation

History and Physical Examination

Identifying Data: Patient's name; age, race, sex. List the patient's significant medical problems. Name of informant (patient, relative).

Chief Compliant : Reason given by patient for seeking medical care and the duration of the symptom.

History of Present Illness (HPI): Describe the course of the patient's illness, including when it began, character of the symptoms, location where the symptoms began; aggravating or alleviating factors; pertinent positives and negatives. Describe past illnesses or surgeries, and past diagnostic testing.

Past Medical History (PMH): Past diseases, surgeries, hospitalizations; medical problems; history of diabetes, hypertension, peptic ulcer disease, asthma, myocardial infarction, cancer. In children include birth history, prenatal history, immunizations, and type of feedings.

Medications:

Allergies: Penicillin, codeine?

Family History: Medical problems in family, including the patient's disorder. Asthma, coronary artery disease, heart failure, cancer, tuberculosis.

Social History: Alcohol, smoking, drug usage. Marital status, employment situation. Level of education.

Review of Systems (ROS):

    General: Weight gain or loss, loss of appetite, fever, chills, fatigue, night sweats.

    Skin: Rashes, skin discolorations.

    Head: Headaches, dizziness, masses, seizures.

    Eyes: Visual changes, eye pain.

    Ears: Tinnitus, vertigo, hearing loss.

    Nose: Nose bleeds, discharge, sinus diseases.

    Mouth and Throat: Dental disease, hoarseness, throat pain.

    Respiratory: Cough, shortness of breath, sputum (color).

    Cardiovascular: Chest pain, orthopnea, paroxysmal nocturnal dyspnea; dyspnea on exertion, claudication, edema, valvular disease.

    Gastrointestinal: Dysphagia, abdominal pain, nausea, vomiting, hematemesis, diarrhea, constipation, melena (black tarry stools), hematochezia (bright red blood per rectum).

    Genitourinary: Dysuria, frequency, hesitancy, hematuria, discharge.

    Gynecological: Gravida/para, abortions, last menstrual period (frequency, duration), age of menarche, menopause; dysmenorrhea, contraception, vaginal bleeding, breast masses.

    Endocrine: Polyuria, polydipsia, skin or hair changes, heat intolerance.

    Musculoskeletal: Joint pain or swelling, arthritis, myalgias.

    Skin and Lymphatics: Easy bruising, lymphadenopathy.

    Neuropsychiatric: Weakness, seizures, memory changes, depression.

Physical Examination

General appearance: Note whether the patient looks "ill," well, or malnourished.

Vital Signs: Temperature, heart rate, respirations, blood pressure.

Skin: Rashes, scars, moles, capillary refill (in seconds).

Lymph Nodes: Cervical, supraclavicular, axillary, inguinal nodes; size, tenderness.

Head: Bruising, masses. Check fontanels in pediatric patients.

Eyes: Pupils equal round and react to light and accommodation (PERRLA); extra ocular movements intact (EOMI), and visual fields. Funduscopy (papilledema, arteriovenous nicking, hemorrhages, exudates); scleral icterus, ptosis.

Ears: Acuity, tympanic membranes (dull, shiny, intact, injected, bulging).

Mouth and Throat: Mucus membrane color and moisture; oral lesions, dentition, pharynx, tonsils.

Neck: Jugular venous distention (JVD) at a 45 degree incline, thyromegaly, lymphadenopathy, masses, bruits, abdominojugular reflux.

Chest: Equal expansion, tactile fremitus, percussion, auscultation, rhonchi, crackles, rubs, breath sounds, egophony, whispered pectoriloquy.

Heart: Point of maximal impulse (PMI), thrills (palpable turbulence); regular rate and rhythm (RRR), first and second heart sounds (S1, S2); gallops (S3, S4), murmurs (grade 1-6), pulses (graded 0-2+).

Breast: Dimpling, tenderness, masses, nipple discharge; axillary masses.

Abdomen: Contour (flat, scaphoid, obese, distended); scars, bowel sounds, bruits, tenderness, masses, liver span by percussion; hepatomegaly, splenomegaly; guarding, rebound, percussion note (tympanic), costovertebral angle tenderness (CVAT), suprapubic tenderness.

Genitourinary: Inguinal masses, hernias, scrotum, testicles, varicoceles.

Pelvic Examination: Vaginal mucosa, cervical discharge, uterine size, masses, adnexal masses, ovaries.

Extremities: Joint swelling, range of motion, edema (grade 1-4+); cyanosis, clubbing, edema (CCE); pulses (radial, ulnar, femoral, popliteal, posterior tibial, dorsalis pedis; simultaneous palpation of radial and femoral pulses).

Rectal Examination: Sphincter tone, masses, fissures; test for occult blood, prostate (nodules, tenderness, size).

Neurological: Mental status and affect; gait, strength (graded 0-5); touch sensation, pressure, pain, position and vibration; deep tendon reflexes (biceps, triceps, patellar, ankle; graded 0-4+); Romberg test (ability to stand erect with arms outstretched and eyes closed).

Cranial Nerve Examination:

    I: Smell

    II: Vision and visual fields

    III, IV, VI: Pupil responses to light, extraocular eye movements, ptosis

    V: Facial sensation, ability to open jaw against resistance, corneal reflex.

    VII: Close eyes tightly, smile, show teeth

    VIII: Hears watch tic; Weber test (lateralization of sound when tuning fork is placed on top of head); Rinne test (air conduction last longer than bone conduction when tuning fork is placed on mastoid process)

    IX, X: Palette moves in midline when patient says "ah," speech

    XI: Shoulder shrug and turns head against resistance

    XII: Stick out tongue in midline

Labs: Electrolytes (sodium, potassium, bicarbonate, chloride, BUN, creatinine), CBC (hemoglobin, hematocrit, WBC count, platelets, differential); x-rays, ECG, urine analysis (UA), liver function tests (LFTs).

Assessment (Impression): Assign a number to each problem and discuss separately. Discuss differential diagnosis and give reasons that support the working diagnosis; give reasons for excluding other diagnoses.

Plan: Describe therapeutic plan for each numbered problem, including testing, laboratory studies, medications, and antibiotics.

Admission Check List

1. **Call and request** old chart, ECG, and X-rays.
2. **Stat labs:** CBC, Chem 7, cardiac enzymes (myoglobin, troponin, CPK), INR, PTT, C&S, ABG, UA.
3. **Labs:** Toxicology screens and drug levels.
4. **Cultures:** Blood culture x 2, urine and sputum culture (before initiating antibiotics), sputum Gram stain, urinalysis.
5. **CXR, ECG**, diagnostic studies.
6. **Discuss case with resident, attending**, and family.

Progress Notes

Daily progress notes should summarize developments in a patient's hospital course, problems that remain active, plans to treat those problems, and arrangements for discharge. Progress notes should address every element of the problem list.

Progress Note

Date/time:
Subjective: Any problems and symptoms of the patient should be charted. Appetite, pain, headaches or insomnia may be included.
Objective:
General appearance.
Vitals, including highest temperature over past 24 hours. Fluid I/O (inputs and outputs), including oral, parenteral, urine, and stool volumes.
Physical exam, including chest and abdomen, with particular attention to active problems. Emphasize changes from previous physical exams.
Labs: Include new test results and circle abnormal values.
Current medications: List all medications and dosages.
Assessment and Plan: This section should be organized by problem. A separate assessment and plan should be written for each problem.

Procedure Note

A procedure note should be written in the chart when a procedure is performed. Procedure notes are brief operative notes.

Procedure Note

Date and time:
Procedure:
Indications:
Patient Consent: Document that the indications and risks were explained to the patient and that the patient consented: "The patient understands the risks of the procedure and consents in writing."
Lab tests: Relevant labs, such as the INR and CBC
Anesthesia: Local with 2% lidocaine
Description of Procedure: Briefly describe the procedure, including sterile prep, anesthesia method, patient position, devices used, anatomic location of procedure, and outcome.
Complications and Estimated Blood Loss (EBL):
Disposition: Describe how the patient tolerated the procedure.
Specimens: Describe any specimens obtained and labs tests which were ordered.

Discharge Note

The discharge note should be written in the patient's chart prior to discharge.

Discharge Note

Date/time:
Diagnoses:
Treatment: Briefly describe treatment provided during hospitalization, including surgical procedures and antibiotic therapy.
Studies Performed: Electrocardiograms, CT scans.
Discharge Medications:
Follow-up Arrangements:

Discharge Summary

Patient's Name and Medical Record Number:
Date of Admission:
Date of Discharge:
Admitting Diagnosis:
Discharge Diagnosis:
Attending or Ward Team Responsible for Patient:
Surgical Procedures, Diagnostic Tests, Invasive Procedures:

Brief History, Pertinent Physical Examination, and Laboratory Data: Describe the course of the patient's disease up until the time that the patient came to the hospital, including physical exam and laboratory data.

Hospital Course: Describe the course of the patient's illness while in the hospital, including evaluation, treatment, medications, and outcome of treatment.

Discharged Condition: Describe improvement or deterioration in the patient's condition, and describe present status of the patient.

Disposition: Describe the situation to which the patient will be discharged (home, nursing home), and indicate who will take care of patient.

Discharged Medications: List medications and instructions for patient on taking the medications.

Discharged Instructions and Follow-up Care: Date of return for follow-up care at clinic; diet, exercise.

Problem List: List all active and past problems.

Copies: Send copies to attending, clinic, consultants.

Prescription Writing

- Patient's name:
- Date:
- Drug name, dosage form, dose, route, frequency (include concentration for oral liquids or mg strength for oral solids): Amoxicillin 125mg/5mL 5 mL PO tid
- Quantity to dispense: mL for oral liquids, # of oral solids
- Refills: If appropriate
- Signature

12 Prescription Writing

Advanced Cardiac Life Support

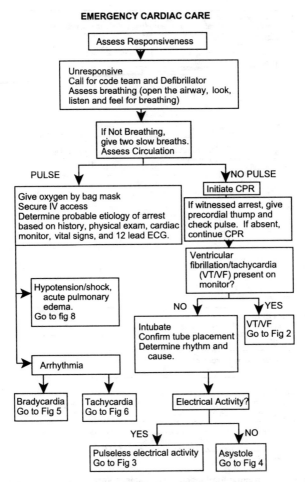

EMERGENCY CARDIAC CARE

Assess Responsiveness

Unresponsive
Call for code team and Defibrillator
Assess breathing (open the airway, look,
listen and feel for breathing)

If Not Breathing,
give two slow breaths.
Assess Circulation

PULSE

Give oxygen by bag mask
Secure IV access
Determine probable etiology of arrest
based on history, physical exam, cardiac
monitor, vital signs, and 12 lead ECG.

NO PULSE

Initiate CPR

If witnessed arrest, give
precordial thump and
check pulse. If absent,
continue CPR

Ventricular
fibrillation/tachycardia
(VT/VF) present on
monitor?

Hypotension/shock,
acute pulmonary
edema.
Go to fig 8

NO

Intubate
Confirm tube placement
Determine rhythm and
cause.

YES

VT/VF
Go to Fig 2

Arrhythmia

Bradycardia
Go to Fig 5

Tachycardia
Go to Fig 6

Electrical Activity?

YES

Pulseless electrical activity
Go to Fig 3

NO

Asystole
Go to Fig 4

Fig 1 - Algorithm for Adult Emergency Cardiac Care

VENTRICULAR FIBRILLATION AND PULSELESS VENTRICULAR TACHYCARDIA

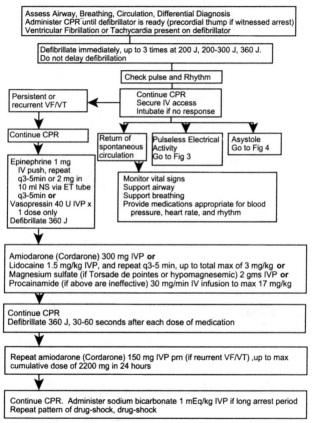

Assess Airway, Breathing, Circulation, Differential Diagnosis
Administer CPR until defibrillator is ready (precordial thump if witnessed arrest)
Ventricular Fibrillation or Tachycardia present on defibrillator

Defibrillate immediately, up to 3 times at 200 J, 200-300 J, 360 J.
Do not delay defibrillation

Check pulse and Rhythm

Continue CPR
Secure IV access
Intubate if no response

Persistent or recurrent VF/VT

Continue CPR

Epinephrine 1 mg
IV push, repeat
q3-5min or 2 mg in
10 ml NS via ET tube
q3-5min or
Vasopressin 40 U IVP x
1 dose only
Defibrillate 360 J

Return of spontaneous circulation

Pulseless Electrical Activity
Go to Fig 3

Asystole
Go to Fig 4

Monitor vital signs
Support airway
Support breathing
Provide medications appropriate for blood
pressure, heart rate, and rhythm

Amiodarone (Cordarone) 300 mg IVP or
Lidocaine 1.5 mg/kg IVP, and repeat q3-5 min, up to total max of 3 mg/kg or
Magnesium sulfate (if Torsade de pointes or hypomagnesemic) 2 gms IVP or
Procainamide (if above are ineffective) 30 mg/min IV infusion to max 17 mg/kg

Continue CPR
Defibrillate 360 J, 30-60 seconds after each dose of medication

Repeat amiodarone (Cordarone) 150 mg IVP prn (if reurrent VF/VT) ,up to max
cumulative dose of 2200 mg in 24 hours

Continue CPR. Administer sodium bicarbonate 1 mEq/kg IVP if long arrest period
Repeat pattern of drug-shock, drug-shock

Note: Epinephrine, lidocaine, atropine may be given via endotracheal tube at
2-2.5 times the IV dose. Dilute in 10 cc of saline.
After each intravenous dose, give 20-30 mL bolus of IV fluid and elevate
extremity.

Fig 2 - Ventricular Fibrillation and Pulseless Ventricular Tachycardia

PULSELESS ELECTRICAL ACTIVITY

Pulseless Electrical Activity Includes:
    Electromechanical dissociation (EMD)
    Pseudo-EMD
    Idioventricular rhythms
    Ventricular escape rhythms
    Bradyasystolic rhythms
    Postdefibrillation idioventricular rhythms

Initiate CPR, secure IV access, intubate, assess pulse.

Determine differential diagnosis and treat underlying cause:
    Hypoxia (ventilate)
    Hypovolemia (infuse volume)
    Pericardial tamponade (performpericardiocentesis)
    Tension pneumothorax (perform needle decompression)
    Pulmonary embolism (thrombectomy, thrombolytics)
    Drug overdose with tricyclics, digoxin, beta, or calcium blockers
    Hyperkalemia or hypokalemia
    Acidosis (give bicarbonate)
    Myocardial infarction (thrombolytics)
    Hypothemia (active rewarming)

Epinephrine 1.0 mg IV bolus q3-5 min, or high dose
    epinephrine 0.1 mg/kg IV push q3-5 min; may give via
    ET tube.
Continue CPR

If bradycardia (<60 beats/min), give atroprine 1 mg IV, q3-5
    min, up to total of 0.04 mg/kg
Consider bicarbonate, 1 mEq/kg IV (1-2 amp, 44 mEq/amp),
    if hyperkalemia or other indications.

Fig 3 - Pulseless Electrical Activity

ASYSTOLE

Continue CPR. Confirm asystole by repositioning paddles or by checking 2 leads. Intubate and secure IV access.

↓

Consider underlying cause, such as hypoxia, hyperkalemia, hypokalemia, acidosis, drug overdose, hypothermia. myocardial infarction.

↓

Consider transcutaneous pacing (TCP)

↓

Epinephrine 1.0 mg IV push, repeat every 3-5 min; may give by ET tube; high dose epinephrine 0.1 mg/kg IV push q5min (1:1000 sln).

↓

Atropine 1 mg IV, repeat q3-5min up to a total of 0.04 mg/kg; may give via ET tube.

↓

Consider bicarbonate 1 mEq/kg (1-2 amp) if hyperkalemia, acidosis, tricyclic overdose. Consider termination of efforts.

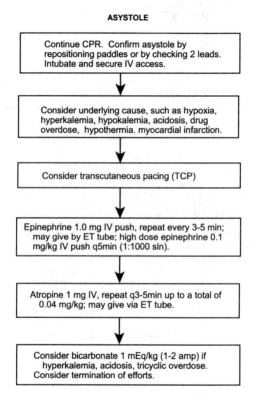

Fig 4 - Asystole

BRADYCARDIA

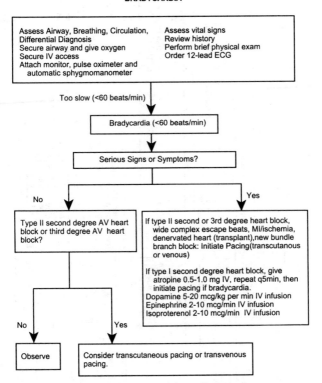

Fig 5 - Bradycardia (with patient not in cardiac arrest).

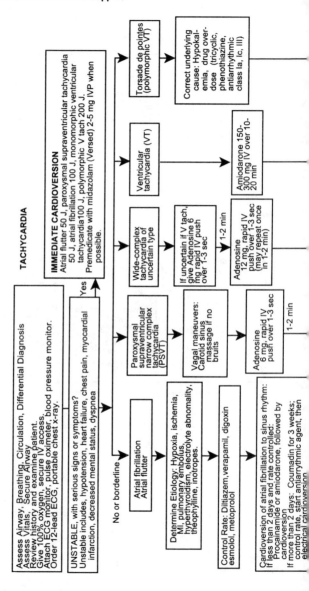

TACHYCARDIA

Assess Airway, Breathing, Circulation, Differential Diagnosis
Assess Vitals, Secure Airway.
Review history and examine patient.
Give 100% oxygen, secure IV access.
Attach ECG monitor, pulse oximeter, blood pressure monitor.
Order 12-lead ECG, portable chest x-ray.

UNSTABLE, with serious signs or symptoms?
Unstable includes, hypotension, heart failure, chest pain, myocardial infarction, decreased mental status, dyspnea

Yes →

IMMEDIATE CARDIOVERSION
Atrial flutter 50 J, paroxysmal supraventricular tachycardia 50 J, atrial fibrillation 100 J, monomorphic ventricular tachycardia 100 J, polymorphic V tach 200 J. Premedicate with midazolam (Versed) 2-5 mg IVP when possible.

No or borderline ↓

Atrial fibrillation / Atrial flutter

Determine Etiology: Hypoxia, ischemia, MI, pulmonary embolus, hyperthyroidism, electrolyte abnormality, theophylline, inotropes.

Control Rate: Diltiazem, verapamil, digoxin, esmolol, metoprolol

Cardioversion of atrial fibrillation to sinus rhythm:
If less than 2 days and rate controlled: Procainamide or amiodarone, followed by cardioversion
If more than 2 days: Coumadin for 3 weeks; control rate, start antiarrhythmic agent, then electrical cardioversion

Paroxysmal supraventricular narrow complex tachycardia (PSVT)

Vagal maneuvers: Carotid sinus massage if no bruits

Adenosine 6 mg, rapid IV push over 1-3 sec

1-2 min

Wide-complex tachycardia of uncertain type

If uncertain if V tach, give Adenosine 6 mg rapid IV push over 1-3 sec

1-2 min

Adenosine 12 mg, rapid IV push over 1-3 sec (may repeat once in 1-2 min)

Ventricular tachycardia (VT)

Amiodarone 150-300 mg IV over 10-20 min

Torsade de pointes (polymorphic VT)

Correct underlying cause: Hypokalemia, drug overdose (tricyclic, phenothiazine, antiarrhythmic class Ia, Ic, III)

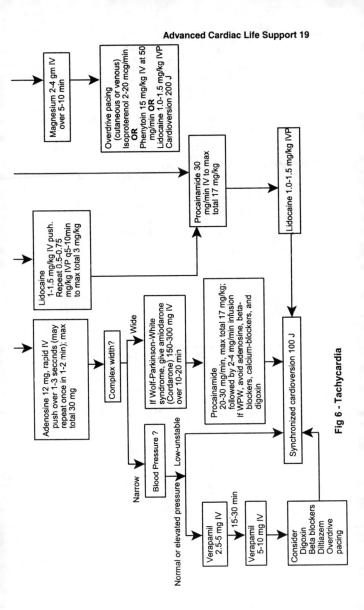

Magnesium 2-4 gm IV over 5-10 min

Overdrive pacing (cutaneous or venous) Isoproterenol 2-20 mcg/min **OR** Phenytoin 15 mg/kg IV at 50 mg/min **OR** Lidocaine 1.0-1.5 mg/kg IVP Cardioversion 200 J

Procainamide 30 mg/min IV to max total 17 mg/kg

Lidocaine 1.0-1.5 mg/kg IVP

Lidocaine 1-1.5 mg/kg IV push. Repeat 0.5-0.75 mg/kg IVP q5-10min to max total 3 mg/kg

Adenosine 12 mg, rapid IV push over 1-3 seconds (may repeat once in 1-2 min); max total 30 mg

Complex width?

Wide

If Wolf-Parkinson-White syndrome, give amiodarone (Cordarone) 150-300 mg IV over 10-20 min

Procainamide 20-30 mg/min, max total 17 mg/kg; followed by 2-4 mg/min infusion If WPW, avoid adenosine, beta-blockers, calcium-blockers, and digoxin

Synchronized cardioversion 100 J

Narrow

Blood Pressure ?

Low-unstable

Normal or elevated pressure

Verapamil 2.5-5 mg IV

15-30 min

Verapamil 5-10 mg IV

Consider Digoxin Beta blockers Diltiazem Overdrive pacing

Fig 6 - Tachycardia

STABLE TACHYCARDIA

Stable tachycardia with serious signs and symptoms related to the tachycardia. Patient not in cardiac arrest.

If ventricular rate is >150 beats/min, prepare for immediate cardioversion. **Treatment of Stable Patients is based on Arrhythmia Type:**

Ventricular Tachycardia:
  Procainamide (Pronestyl) 30 mg/min IV, up to a total max of 17 mg/kg, or
  Amiodarone (Cordarone) 150-300 mg IV over 10-20 min, or
  Lidocaine 0.75 mg/kg. Procainamide should be avoided if ejection fraction is <40%.

Paroxysmal Supraventricular Tachycardia: Carotid sinus pressure (if bruits absent), then adenosine 6 mg rapid IVP, followed by 12 mg rapid IVP x 2 doses to max total 30 mg. If no response, verapamil 2.5-5.0 mg IVP; may repeat dose with 5-10 mg IVP if adequate blood pressure; or Esmolol 500 mcg/kg IV over 1 min, then 50 mcg/kg/min IV infusion, and titrate up to 200 mcg/kg/min IV infusion.

Atrial Fibrillation/Flutter:
  Ejection fraction ≥40%: Diltiazem (Cardiazem) 0.25 mg/kg IV over 2 min; may repeat 0.35 mg/kg IV over 2 min prn x 1 to control rate. Then give procainamide (Pronestyl) 30 mg/min IV infusion, up to a total max of 17 mg/kg
  Ejection fraction <40%: Digoxin 0.5 mg IVP, then 0.25 mg IVP q4h x 2 to control rate. Then give amiodarone (Cordarone) 150-300 mg IV over 10-20 min.

Check oxygen saturation, suction device, intubation equipment. Secure IV access

Premedicate whenever possible with Midazolam (Versed) 2-5 mg IVP or sodium pentothal 2 mg/kg rapid IVP

Synchronized cardioversion	
Atrialflutter	50 J
PSVT	50 J
Atrial	100 J
Monomorphic V-tach	100 J
Polymorphic V tach	200 J

Fig 7 - Stable Tachycardia (not in cardiac arrest)

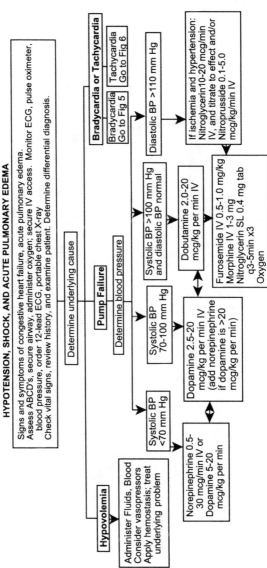

HYPOTENSION, SHOCK, AND ACUTE PULMONARY EDEMA

Signs and symptoms of congestive heart failure, acute pulmonary edema.
Assess ABCD's, secure airway, administer oxygen; secure IV access. Monitor ECG, pulse oximeter, blood pressure, order 12-lead ECG, portable chest X-ray
Check vital signs, review history, and examine patient. Determine differential diagnosis.

Determine underlying cause

Hypovolemia

Administer Fluids, Blood
Consider vasopressors
Apply hemostasis; treat underlying problem

Pump Failure

Determine blood pressure

Systolic BP
<70 mm Hg

Norepinephrine 0.5-30 mcg/min IV or Dopamine 5-20 mcg/kg per min

Systolic BP
70-100 mm Hg

Dopamine 2.5-20 mcg/kg per min IV (add norepinephrine if dopamine is >20 mcg/kg per min)

Systolic BP >100 mm Hg and diastolic BP normal

Dobutamine 2.0-20 mcg/kg per min IV

Bradycardia or Tachycardia

Bradycardia
Go to Fig 5

Tachycardia
Go to Fig 6

Diastolic BP >110 mm Hg

If ischemia and hypertension:
Nitroglycerin 10-20 mcg/min IV, and titrate to effect and/or Nitroprusside 0.1-5.0 mcg/kg/min IV

Furosemide IV 0.5-1.0 mg/kg
Morphine IV 1-3 mg
Nitroglycerin SL 0.4 mg tab q3-5min x3
Oxygen

Fig 8 - Hypotension, Shock, and Acute Pulmonary Edema

Cardiovascular Disorders

ST-Segment Elevation Myocardial Infarction

1. **Admit to:** Coronary care unit
2. **Diagnosis:** Rule out myocardial infarction
3. **Condition:**
4. **Vital Signs:** q1h. Call physician if pulse >90,<60; BP >150/90, <90/60; R>25, <12; T >38.5°C.
5. **Activity:** Bed rest with bedside commode.
7. **Nursing:** Guaiac stools. If patient has chest pain, obtain 12-lead ECG and call physician.
8. **Diet:** Cardiac diet, 1-2 gm sodium, low fat, low cholesterol diet. No caffeine or temperature extremes.
9. **IV Fluids:** D5W at TKO
10. **Special Medications:**
    -Oxygen 2-4 L/min by NC.
    -Aspirin 325 mg PO, chew and swallow, then aspirin EC 162 mg PO qd **OR** Clopidogrel (Plavix) 75 mg PO qd (if allergic to aspirin).
    -Nitroglycerine 10 mcg/min infusion (50 mg in 250-500 mL D5W, 100-200 mcg/mL). Titrate to control symptoms in 5-10 mcg/min steps, up to 200-300 mcg/min; maintain systolic BP >90 **OR**
    -Nitroglycerine SL, 0.4 mg (0.15-0.6 mg) SL q5min until pain free (up to 3 tabs) **OR**
    -Nitroglycerin spray (0.4 mg/aerosol spray)1-2 sprays under the tongue q 5min; may repeat x 2.
    -Heparin 60 U/kg IV push, then 12 U/kg/hr by continuous IV infusion for 48 hours to maintain aPTT of 50-70 seconds. Check aPTTq6h x 4, then qd. Repeat aPTT 6 hours after each heparin dosage change.

Thrombolytic Therapy

Absolute Contraindications to Thrombolytics: Active internal bleeding, suspected aortic dissection, known intracranial neoplasm, previous intracranial hemorrhagic stroke at any time, other strokes or cerebrovascular events within 1 year, head trauma, pregnancy, recent non-compressible vascular puncture, uncontrolled hypertension (>180/110 mmHg).

Relative Contraindications to Thrombolytics: Absence of ST-segment elevation, severe hypertension, cerebrovascular disease, recent surgery (within 2 weeks), cardiopulmonary resuscitation.

A. Alteplase (tPA, tissue plasminogen activator, Activase):
1. 15 mg IV push over 2 min, followed by 0.75 mg/kg (max 50 mg) IV infusion over 30 min, followed by 0.5 mg/kg (max 35 mg) IV infusion over 60 min (max total dose 100 mg).
2. **Labs:** INR/PTT, CBC, fibrinogen.

B. Reteplase (Retavase):
1. 10 U IV push over 2 min; repeat second 10 U IV push after 30 min.
2. **Labs:** INR, aPTT, CBC, fibrinogen.

C. Tenecteplase (TNKase):

<60 kg	30 mg IVP
60-69 kg	35 mg IVP
70-79 kg	40 mg IVP

80-89 kg	45 mg IVP
≥90 kg	50 mg IVP

C. Streptokinase (Streptase):
   1. 1.5 million IU in 100 mL NS IV over 60 min. Pretreat with diphenhydramine (Benadryl) 50 mg IV push **AND**
      Methylprednisolone (Soln-Medrol) 250 mg IV push.
   2. Check fibrinogen level now and q6h for 24h until level >100 mg/dL.
   3. No IM or arterial punctures, watch IV for bleeding.

Angiotensin Converting Enzyme Inhibitor:
   -Lisinopril (Zestril, Prinivil) 2.5-5 mg PO qd; titrate to 10-20 mg qd.

Long-acting Nitrates:
   -Nitroglycerin patch 0.2 mg/hr qd. Allow for nitrate-free period to prevent tachyphylaxis.
   -Isosorbide dinitrate (Isordil) 10-60 mg PO tid [5,10,20, 30,40 mg] **OR**
   -Isosorbide mononitrate (Imdur) 30-60 mg PO qd.

Beta-Blockers: Contraindicated in cardiogenic shock.
   -Metoprolol (Lopressor) 5 mg IV q2-5min x 3 doses; then 25 mg PO q6h for 48h, then 100 mg PO q12h; hold if heart rate <60/min or systolic BP <100 mmHg **OR**
   -Atenolol (Tenormin), 5 mg IV, repeated in 5 minutes, followed by 50-100 mg PO qd **OR**
   -Esmolol hydrochloride (Brevibloc) 500 mcg/kg IV over 1 min, then 50 mcg/kg/min IV infusion, titrated to heart rate >60 bpm (max 300 mcg/kg/min).

Statins:
   -Atorvastatin (Lipitor) 10 mg PO qhs **OR**
   -Pravastatin (Pravachol) 40 mg PO qhs **OR**
   -Simvastatin (Zocor) 20 mg PO qhs **OR**
   -Lovastatin (Mevacor) 20 mg PO qhs **OR**
   -Fluvastatin (Lescol)10-20 mg PO qhs.

11. **Symptomatic Medications:**
    -Morphine sulfate 2-4 mg IV push prn chest pain.
    -Acetaminophen (Tylenol) 325-650 mg PO q4-6h prn headache.
    -Lorazepam (Ativan) 1-2 mg PO tid-qid prn anxiety
    -Zolpidem (Ambien) 5-10 mg qhs prn insomnia.
    -Docusate (Colace) 100 mg PO bid.
    -Dimenhydrinate (Dramamine) 25-50 mg IV over 2-5 min q4-6h or 50 mg PO q4-6h prn nausea.
    -Famotidine (Pepcid) 20 mg IV/PO bid.

12. **Extras:** ECG stat and in 12h and in AM, portable CXR, impedance cardiography, echocardiogram. Cardiology consult.

13. **Labs:** SMA7 and 12, magnesium. Cardiac enzymes: CPK-MB, troponin T, myoglobin STAT and q6h for 24h. CBC, INR/PTT, UA.

Non-ST Segment Elevation Myocardial Infarction (NSTEMI)

1. **Admit to:** Coronary care unit
2. **Diagnosis:** Unstable Angina
3 **Condition:**
4. **Vital Signs:** q1h. Call physician if pulse >90,<60; BP >150/90, <90/60; R>25, <12; T >38.5°C.
5. **Activity:** Bed rest with bedside commode.
7. **Nursing:** Guaiac stools. If patient has chest pain, obtain 12-lead ECG and call physician.
8. **Diet:** Cardiac diet, 1-2 gm sodium, low fat, low cholesterol diet. No caffeine or temperature extremes.
9. **IV Fluids:** D5W at TKO
10. **Special Medications:**
    -Oxygen 2-4 L/min by NC.
    -Aspirin 325 mg PO, chew and swallow, then aspirin EC 162 mg PO qd **OR**
    -Clopidogrel (Plavix) 75 mg PO qd (if allergic to aspirin).
    -Nitroglycerine infusion 10 mcg/min infusion (50 mg in 250-500 mL D5W, 100-200 mcg/mL). Titrate to control symptoms in 5-10 mcg/min steps, up to 200-300 mcg/min; maintain systolic BP >90 **OR**
    -Nitroglycerine SL, 0.4 mg (0.15-0.6 mg) SL q5min until pain free (up to 3 tabs) **OR**
    -Nitroglycerin spray (0.4 mg/aerosol spray)1-2 sprays under the tongue q 5min; MR x 2.
    -Heparin 60 U/kg IV push, then 12 U/kg/hr by continuous IV infusion for 48 hours to maintain aPTT of 50-70 seconds. Check aPTTq6h x 4, then qd. Repeat aPTT 6 hours after each heparin dosage change.

Glycoprotein II$_b$/III$_a$ Blockers:
    -Eptifibatide (Integrilin) 180mcg/kg IVP, then 2 mcg/kg/min for 72 hours **OR**
    -Tirofiban (Aggrastat) 0.4 mcg/kg/min for 30 min, then 0.1 mcg/kg/min for 48-108 hours.

Glycoprotein IIb/IIIa blockers for Use With Angioplasty:
    -Abciximab (ReoPro) 0.25 mg/kg IVP, then 0.125 mcg/kg/min IV infusion for 12 hours **OR**
    -Eptifibatide (Integrilin) 180 mcg/kg IVP, then 2 mcg/kg/min for 20-24 hours.

Angiotensin Converting Enzyme Inhibitor:
    -Lisinopril (Zestril, Prinivil) 2.5-5 mg PO qd; titrate to 10-20 mg qd.

Long-acting Nitrates:
    -Nitroglycerin patch 0.2 mg/hr qd. Allow for nitrate-free period to prevent tachyphylaxis.
    -Isosorbide dinitrate (Isordil) 10-60 mg PO tid [5,10,20, 30,40 mg] **OR**
    -Isosorbide mononitrate (Imdur) 30-60 mg PO qd.

Beta-Blockers: Contraindicated in cardiogenic shock.
    -Metoprolol (Lopressor) 5 mg IV q2-5min x 3 doses; then 25 mg PO q6h for 48h, then 100 mg PO q12h; keep HR <60/min, hold if systolic BP <100 mmHg **OR**
    -Atenolol (Tenormin), 5 mg IV, repeated in 5 minutes, followed by 50-100 mg PO qd **OR**
    -Esmolol (Brevibloc) 500 mcg/kg IV over 1 min, then 50 mcg/kg/min IV

infusion, titrated to heart rate >60 bpm (max 300 mcg/kg/min).

Statins:
- -Atorvastatin (Lipitor) 10 mg PO qhs **OR**
- -Pravastatin (Pravachol) 40 mg PO qhs **OR**
- -Simvastatin (Zocor) 20 mg PO qhs **OR**
- -Lovastatin (Mevacor) 20 mg PO qhs **OR**
- -Fluvastatin (Lescol)10-20 mg PO qhs.

11. Symptomatic Medications:
- -Morphine sulfate 2-4 mg IV push prn chest pain.
- -Acetaminophen (Tylenol) 325-650 mg PO q4-6h prn headache.
- -Lorazepam (Ativan) 1-2 mg PO tid-qid prn anxiety.
- -Zolpidem (Ambien) 5-10 mg qhs prn insomnia.
- -Docusate (Colace) 100 mg PO bid.
- -Dimenhydrinate (Dramamine) 25-50 mg IV over 2-5 min q4-6h or 50 mg PO q4-6h prn nausea.
- -Famotidine (Pepcid) 20 mg IV/PO bid.

12. Extras: ECG stat and in 12h and in AM, portable CXR, impedance cardiography, echocardiogram. Cardiology consult.

13. Labs: SMA7 and 12, magnesium. Cardiac enzymes: CPK-MB, troponin T, myoglobin STAT and q6h for 24h. CBC, INR/PTT, UA.

Congestive Heart Failure

1. Admit to:

2. Diagnosis: Congestive Heart Failure

3. Condition:

4. Vital Signs: q1h. Call physician if P >120; BP >150/100 <80/60; T >38.5°C; R >25, <10.

5. Activity: Bed rest with bedside commode.

6. Nursing: Daily weights, measure inputs and outputs. Head-of-bed at 45 degrees, legs elevated.

7. Diet: 1-2 gm salt, cardiac diet.

8. IV Fluids: Heparin lock with flush q shift.

9. Special Medications:
- -Oxygen 2-4 L/min by NC.

Diuretics:
- -Furosemide (Lasix) 10-160 mg IV qd-bid or 20-80 mg PO qAM-bid [20,40,80 mg] or 10-40 mg/hr IV infusion **OR**
- -Torsemide (Demadex) 10-40 mg IV or PO qd; max 200 mg/day [5, 10, 20, 100 mg] **OR**
- -Bumetanide (Bumex) 0.5-1 mg IV q2-3h until response; then 0.5-1.0 mg IV q8-24h (max 10 mg/d); or 0.5-2.0 mg PO qAM.
- -Metolazone (Zaroxolyn) 2.5-10 mg PO qd, max 20 mg/d; 30 min before loop diuretic [2.5,5,10 mg].

ACE Inhibitors:
- -Quinapril (Accupril) 5-10 mg PO qd x 1 dose, then 20-80 mg PO qd in 1 to 2 divided doses [5,10,20,40 mg] **OR**
- -Lisinopril (Zestril, Prinivil) 5-40 mg PO qd [5,10,20,40 mg] **OR**
- -Benazepril (Lotensin) 10-20 mg PO qd-bid, max 80 mg/d [5,10,20,40 mg] **OR**
- -Fosinopril (Monopril) 10-40 mg PO qd, max 80 mg/d [10,20 mg] **OR**
- -Ramipril (Altace) 2.5-10 mg PO qd, max 20 mg/d [1.25,2.5,5,10 mg].

-Captopril (Capoten) 6.25-50 mg PO q8h [12.5, 25,50,100 mg] **OR**
-Enalapril (Vasotec) 1.25-5 mg slow IV push q6h or 2.5-20 mg PO bid [5,10,20 mg] **OR**
-Moexipril (Univasc) 7.5 mg PO qd x 1 dose, then 7.5-15 mg PO qd-bid [7.5, 15 mg tabs] **OR**
-Trandolapril (Mavik) 1 mg qd x 1 dose, then 2-4 mg qd [1, 2, 4 mg tabs].

Angiotensin-II Receptor Blockers:
-Irbesartan (Avapro) 150 mg qd, max 300 mg qd [75, 150, 300 mg].
-Losartan (Cozaar) 25-50 mg bid [25, 50 mg].
-Valsartan (Diovan) 80 mg qd; max 320 mg qd [80, 160 mg].
-Candesartan (Atacand) 8-16 mg qd-bid [4, 8, 16, 32 mg].
-Telmisartan (Micardis) 40-80 mg qd [40, 80 mg].

Beta-blockers:
-Carvedilol (Coreg) 1.625-3.125 mg PO bid, then slowly increase the dose every 2 weeks to target dose of 25-50 mg bid [tab 3.125, 6.25, 12.5, 25 mg] **OR**
-Metoprolol (Lopressor) start at 12.5 mg bid, then slowly increase to target dose of 100 mg bid [50, 100 mg].
-Bisoprolol (Zebeta) start at 1.25 mg qd, then slowly increase to target of 10 mg qd. [5,10 mg].

Digoxin: (Lanoxin) 0.125-0.5 mg PO or IV qd [0.125,0.25, 0.5 mg].

Inotropic Agents:
-Dobutamine (Dobutrex) 2.5-10 mcg/kg/min IV, max of 14 mcg/kg/min (500 mg in 250 mL D5W, 2 mg/mL) **OR**
-Dopamine (Intropin) 3-15 mcg/kg/min IV (400 mg in 250 cc D5W, 1600 mcg/mL), titrate to CO >4, CI >2; systolic >90 **OR**
-Milrinone (Primacor) 0.375 mcg/kg/min IV infusion (40 mg in 200 mL NS, 0.2 mg/mL); titrate to 0.75 mgc/kg/min; arrhythmogenic; may cause hypotension.

Vasodilators:
-Nitroglycerin 5 mcg/min IV infusion (50 mg in 250 mL D5W). Titrate in increments of 5 mcg/min to control symptoms and maintain systolic BP >90 mmHg.
-Nesiritide (Natrecor) 2 mcg/kg IV load over 1 min, then 0.010 mcg/kg/min IV infusion. Titrate in increments of 0.005 mcg/kg/min q3h to max 0.03 mcg/kg/min IV infusion.

Potassium:
-KCL (Micro-K) 20-60 mEq PO qd if the patient is taking loop diuretics.

Pacing:
-Synchronized biventricular pacing if ejection fraction <40% and QRS duration >150 msec.

10. Symptomatic Medications:
-Morphine sulfate 2-4 mg IV push prn dyspnea or anxiety.
-Heparin 5000 U SQ q12h or enoxaparin (Lovenox) 1 mg/kg SC q12h.
-Docusate sodium (Colace) 100-200 mg PO qhs.
-Famotidine (Pepcid) 20 mg IV/PO q12h.

11. Extras: CXR PA and LAT, ECG now and repeat if chest pain or palpitations, impedance cardiography, echocardiogram.

12. Labs: SMA 7&12, CBC; B-type natriuretic peptide (BNP), cardiac enzymes: CPK-MB, troponin T, myoglobin STAT and q6h for 24h. Repeat SMA 7 in AM. UA.

Supraventricular Tachycardia

1. **Admit to:**
2. **Diagnosis:** PSVT
3. **Condition:**
4. **Vital Signs:** q1h. Call physician if BP >160/90, <90/60; apical pulse >130, <50; R >25, <10; T >38.5°C
5. **Activity:** Bedrest with bedside commode.
6. **Nursing:**
7. **Diet:** Low fat, low cholesterol, no caffeine.
8. **IV Fluids:** D5W at TKO.
9. **Special Medications:**
   Attempt vagal maneuvers (Valsalva maneuver) before drug therapy.
   Cardioversion (if unstable or refractory to drug therapy):
   1. NPO for 6h, digoxin level must be less than 2.4 and potassium and magnesium must be normal.
   2. Midazolam (Versed) 2-5 mg IV push.
   3. If stable, cardiovert with synchronized 10-50 J, and increase by 50 J increments if necessary. If unstable, start with 75-100 J, then increase to 200 J and 360 J.

   Pharmacologic Therapy of Supraventricular Tachycardia:
   -Adenosine (Adenocard) 6 mg rapid IV over 1-2 sec, followed by saline flush, may repeat 12 mg IV after 2-3 min, to max of 30 mg total **OR**
   -Verapamil (Isoptin) 2.5-5 mg IV over 2-3min (may give calcium gluconate 1 gm IV over 3-6 min prior to verapamil); then 40-120 mg PO q8h [40, 80, 120 mg] or verapamil SR 120-240 mg PO qd [120, 180, 240 mg] **OR**
   -Esmolol hydrochloride (Brevibloc) 500 mcg/kg IV over 1 min, then 50 mcg/kg/min IV infusion titrated to HR of <80 (max of 300 mcg/kg/min) **OR**
   -Diltiazem (Cardizem) 0.25 mg/kg IV over 2-5 minutes, followed by 5 mg/h IV infusion. Titrate to max 15 mg/h; then diltiazem-CD (Cardizem-CD)120-240 mg PO qd **OR**
   -Metoprolol (Lopressor) 5 mg IVP q4-6h; then 50-100 mg PO bid, or metoprolol XL (Toprol-XL) 50-100 mg PO qd **OR**
   -Digoxin (Lanoxin) 0.25 mg q4h as needed; up to 1.0-1.5 mg; then 0.125-0.25 mg PO qd.
10. **Symptomatic Medications:**
    -Lorazepam (Ativan) 1-2 mg PO tid prn anxiety.
11. **Extras:** Portable CXR, ECG; repeat if chest pain. Cardiology consult.
12. **Labs:** CBC, SMA 7&12, Mg, thyroid panel. UA.

Ventricular Arrhythmias

1. **Ventricular Fibrillation and Tachycardia:**
   -**If unstable (see ACLS protocol):** Defibrillate with unsynchronized 200 J, then 300 J.
   -Oxygen 100% by mask.
   -Lidocaine (Xylocaine) loading dose 75-100 mg IV, then 2-4 mg/min IV **OR**
   -Amiodarone (Cordarone) 300 mg in 100 mL of D5W, IV infusion over 10 min, then 900 mg in 500 mL of D5W, at 1 mg/min for 6 hrs, then at 0.5 mg/min thereafter; or 400 mg PO q8h x 14 days, then 200-400 mg qd.

-**Also see "other antiarrhythmics" below.**
2. **Torsades De Pointes Ventricular Tachycardia:**
   -Correct underlying cause and consider discontinuing quinidine, procainamide, disopyramide, moricizine, amiodarone, sotalol, Ibutilide,
   phenothiazine, haloperidol, tricyclic and tetracyclic antidepressants,
   ketoconazole, itraconazole, bepridil, hypokalemia, and hypomagnesemia.
   -Magnesium sulfate 1-4 gm in IV bolus over 5-15 min or infuse 3-20 mg/min
   for 7-48h until QTc interval <440 msec.
   -Isoproterenol (Isuprel), 2-20 mcg/min (2 mg in 500 mL D5W, 4 mcg/mL).
   -Consider ventricular pacing and/or cardioversion.
3. **Other Antiarrhythmics:**
   Class I:
   -Moricizine (Ethmozine) 200-300 mg PO q8h, max 900 mg/d [200, 250, 300
   mg].
   Class Ia:
   -Quinidine gluconate (Quinaglute) 324-648 mg PO q8-12h [324 mg].
   -Procainamide (Procan, Procanbid)
       IV: 15 mg/kg IV loading dose at 20 mg/min, followed by 2-4 mg/min
       continuous IV infusion.
       PO: 500 mg (nonsustained release) PO q2h x 2 doses, then Procanbid 1-
       2 gm PO q12h [500, 1000 mg].
   -Disopyramide (Nor-pace, Norpace CR) 100-300 mg PO q6-8h [100, 150, mg]
   or disopyramide CR 100-150 mg PO bid [100, 150 mg].
   Class Ib:
   -Lidocaine (Xylocaine) 75-100 mg IV, then 2-4 mg/min IV
   -Mexiletine (Mexitil) 100-200 mg PO q8h, max 1200 mg/d [150, 200, 250 mg].
   -Tocainide (Tonocard) loading 400-600 mg PO, then 400-600 mg PO q8-12h
   (1200-1800 mg/d) PO in divided doses q8-12h [400, 600 mg].
   -Phenytoin (Dilantin), loading dose 100-300 mg IV given as 50 mg in NS over
   10 min IV q5min, then 100 mg IV q5min prn.
   Class Ic:
   -Flecainide (Tambocor) 50-100 mg PO q12h, max 400 mg/d [50, 100, 150
   mg].
   -Propafenone (Rythmol) 150-300 mg PO q8h, max 1200 mg/d [150, 225, 300
   mg].
   Class II:
   -Propranolol (Inderal) 1-3 mg IV in NS (max 0.15 mg/kg) or 20-80 mg PO tid-
   qid [10, 20, 40, 60, 80 mg]; propranolol-LA (Inderal-LA), 80-120 mg PO qd
   [60, 80, 120, 160 mg]
   -Esmolol (Brevibloc) loading dose 500 mcg/kg over 1 min, then 50-200
   mcg/kg/min IV infusion
   -Atenolol (Tenormin) 50-100 mg/d PO [25, 50, 100 mg].
   -Nadolol (Corgard) 40-100 mg PO qd-bid [20, 40, 80, 120, 160 mg].
   -Metoprolol (Lopressor) 50-100 mg PO bid-tid [50, 100 mg], or metoprolol XL
   (Toprol-XL) 50-200 mg PO qd [50, 100, 200 mg].
   Class III:
   -Amiodarone (Cordarone), PO loading 400-1200 mg/d in divided doses for 2-
   4 weeks, then 200-400 mg PO qd (5-10 mg/kg) [200 mg] or amiodarone
   (Cordarone) 300 mg in 100 mL of D5W, IV infusion over 10-20 min, then
   900 mg in 500 mL of D5W, at 1 mg/min for 6 hrs, then at 0.5 mg/min
   thereafter.
   -Sotalol (Betapace) 40-80 mg PO bid, max 320 mg/d in 2-3 divided doses [80,
   160 mg].

4. **Extras:** CXR, ECG, Holter monitor, signal averaged ECG, cardiology consult.
5. **Labs:** SMA 7&12, Mg, calcium, CBC, drug levels. UA.

Hypertensive Emergency

1. **Admit to:**
2. **Diagnosis:** Hypertensive emergency
3. **Condition:**
4. **Vital Signs:** q30min until BP controlled, then q4h.
5. **Activity:** Bed rest
6. **Nursing:** Intra-arterial BP monitoring, daily weights, inputs and outputs.
7. **Diet:** Clear liquids.
8. **IV Fluids:** D5W at TKO.
9. **Special Medications:**
    -Nitroprusside sodium 0.25-10 mcg/kg/min IV (50 mg in 250 mL of D5W), titrate to desired BP
    -Labetalol (Trandate, Normodyne) 20 mg IV bolus (0.25 mg/kg), then 20-80 mg boluses IV q10-15min titrate to desired BP or continuous IV infusion of 1.0-2.0 mg/min titrate to desired BP. Ideal in patients with an aortic aneurysm.
    -Fenoldopam (Corlopam) 0.01mcg/kg/min IV infusion. Adjust dose by 0.025-0.05 mcg/kg/min q15min to max 0.3 mcg/kg/min. [10 mg in 250 mL D5W].
    -Nicardipine (Cardene IV) 5 mg/hr IV infusion, increase rate by 2.5 mg/hr every 15 min up to 15 mg/hr (25 mg in D5W 250 mL).
    -Enalaprilat (Vasotec IV) 1.25- 5.0 mg IV q6h. Do not use in presence of AMI.
    -Esmolol (Brevibloc) 500 mcg/kg/min IV infusion for 1 minute, then 50 mcg/kg/min; titrate by 50 mcg/kg/min increments to 300 mcg/kg/min (2.5 gm in D5W 250 mL).
    -Clonidine (Catapres), initial 0.1-0.2 mg PO followed by 0.05-0.1 mg per hour until DBP <115 (max total dose of 0.8 mg).
    -Phentolamine (pheochromocytoma), 5-10 mg IV, repeated as needed up to 20 mg.
    -Trimethaphan camsylate (Arfonad)(dissecting aneurysm) 2-4 mg/min IV infusion (500 mg in 500 mL of D5W).
10. **Symptomatic Medications:**
    -Acetaminophen (Tylenol) 325-650 mg PO q4-6h prn headache.
    -Zolpidem (Ambien) 5-10 mg qhs prn insomnia.
    -Docusate sodium (Colace) 100-200 mg PO qhs.
11. **Extras:** Portable CXR, ECG, impedance cardiography, echocardiogram.
12. **Labs:** CBC, SMA 7, UA with micro. TSH, free T4, 24h urine for metanephrine. Plasma catecholamines, urine drug screen.

Hypertension

I. **Initial Diagnostic Evaluation of Hypertension**
    A. **15 Lead electrocardiography** may document evidence of ischemic heart disease, rhythm and conduction disturbances, or left ventricular hypertrophy.
    B. **Screening labs** include a complete blood count, glucose, potassium, calcium, creatinine, BUN, uric acid, and fasting lipid panel.

C. **Urinalysis.** Dipstick testing should include glucose, protein, and hemoglobin.
D. Selected patients may require plasma renin activity, 24 hour urine catecholamines, or renal function testing (glomerular filtration rate and blood flow).

II. **Antihypertensive Drugs**

A. **Thiazide Diuretics**
   1. **Hydrochlorothiazide (HCTZ, HydroDiuril)**, 12.5-25 mg qd [25 mg].
   2. **Chlorothiazide (Diuril)** 250 mg qd [250, 500 mg].
   3. **Thiazide/Potassium Sparing Diuretic Combinations**
      a. **Maxzide** (hydrochlorothiazide 50/triamterene 75 mg) 1 tab qd.
      b. **Moduretic** (hydrochlorothiazide 50 mg/amiloride 5 mg) 1 tab qd.
      c. **Dyazide** (hydrochlorothiazide 25 mg/triamterene 37.5) 1 cap qd.

B. **Beta-Adrenergic Blockers**
   1. **Cardioselective Beta-Blockers**
      a. **Atenolol (Tenormin)** initial dose 50 mg qd, then 50-100 mg qd, max 200 mg/d [25, 50, 100 mg].
      b. **Metoprolol XL (Toprol XL)** 100-200 mg qd [50, 100, 200 mg tab ER].
      c. **Bisoprolol (Zebeta)** 2.5-10 mg qd; max 20 mg qd [5,10 mg].
   2. **Non-Cardioselective Beta-Blockers**
      a. **Propranolol LA (Inderal LA)**, 80-160 mg qd [60, 80, 120, 160 mg].
      b. **Nadolol (Corgard)** 40-80 mg qd, max 320 mg/d [20, 40, 80, 120, 160 mg].
      c. **Pindolol (Visken)** 5-20 mg qd, max 60 mg/d [5, 10 mg].
      d. **Carteolol (Cartrol)** 2.5-10 mg qd [2.5, 5 mg].

C. **Angiotensin-Converting Enzyme (ACE) Inhibitors**
   1. **Ramipril (Altace)** 2.5-10 mg qd, max 20 mg/day [1.25, 2.5, 5, 10 mg].
   2. **Quinapril (Accupril)** 20-80 mg qd [5, 10, 20, 40 mg].
   3. **Lisinopril (Zestril, Prinivil)** 10-40 mg qd [2.5, 5, 10, 20, 40 mg].
   4. **Benazepril (Lotensin)** 10-40 mg qd, max 80 mg/day [5, 10, 20, 40 mg].
   5. **Fosinopril (Monopril)** 10-40 mg qd [10, 20 mg].
   6. **Enalapril (Vasotec)** 5-40 mg qd, max 40 mg/day [2.5, 5, 10, 20 mg].
   7. **Moexipril (Univasc)** 7.5-15 mg qd [7.5 mg].

D. **Angiotensin Receptor Blockers**
   1. **Losartan (Cozaar)** 25-50 mg bid [25, 50 mg].
   2. **Valsartan (Diovan)** 80-160 mg qd; max 320 mg qd [80, 160 mg].
   3. **Irbesartan (Avapro)** 150 mg qd; max 300 mg qd [75, 150, 300 mg].
   4. **Candesartan (Atacand)** 8-16 mg qd-bid [4, 8, 16, 32 mg].
   5. **Telmisartan (Micardis)** 40-80 mg qd [40, 80 mg].

E. **Calcium Entry Blockers**
   1. **Diltiazem SR (Cardizem SR)** 60-120 mg bid [60, 90, 120 mg] or **Cardizem CD** 180-360 mg qd [120, 180, 240, 300 mg].
   2. **Nifedipine XL (Procardia-XL, Adalat-CC)** 30-90 mg qd [30, 60, 90 mg].
   3. **Verapamil SR (Calan SR, Covera-HS)** 120-240 mg qd [120, 180, 240 mg].
   4. **Amlodipine (Norvasc)** 2.5-10 mg qd [2.5, 5, 10 mg].
   5. **Felodipine (Plendil)** 5-10 mg qd [2.5, 5, 10 mg].

Syncope

1. **Admit to:** Monitored ward
2. **Diagnosis:** Syncope
3. **Condition:**
4. **Vital Signs:** q1h, postural BP and pulse q12h. Call physician if BP >160/90, <90/60; P >120, <50; R>25, <10
5. **Activity:** Bed rest.
6. **Nursing:** Fingerstick glucose.
7. **Diet:** Regular
8. **IV Fluids:** Normal saline at TKO.
9. **Special medications:**
High-grade AV Block with Syncope:
    -Atropine 1 mg IV x 2.
    -Isoproterenol 0.5-1 mcg/min initially, then slowly titrate to 10 mcg/min IV infusion (1 mg in 250 mL NS).
    -Transthoracic pacing.
Drug-induced Syncope:
    -Discontinue vasodilators, centrally acting hypotensive agents, tranquilizers, antidepressants, and alcohol use.
Vasovagal Syncope:
    -Scopolamine 1.5 mg transdermal patch q3 days.
Postural Syncope:
    -Midodrine (ProAmatine) 2.5 mg PO tid, then increase to 5-10 mg PO tid [2.5, 5 mg]; contraindicated in coronary artery disease.
    -Fludrocortisone 0.1-1.0 mg PO qd.
10. **Symptomatic Medications:**
    -Acetaminophen (Tylenol) 325-650 mg PO q4-6h prn headache.
    -Docusate sodium (Colace) 100-200 mg PO qhs.
11. **Extras:** CXR, ECG, 24h Holter monitor, electrophysiologic study, tilt test, CT/MRI, EEG, impedance cardiography, echocardiogram.
12. **Labs:** CBC, SMA 7&12, CK-MB, troponin T, Mg, calcium, drug levels. UA, urine drug screen.

Pulmonary Disorders

Asthma

1. **Admit to:**
2. **Diagnosis:** Exacerbation of asthma
3. **Condition:**
4. **Vital Signs:** q6h. Call physician if P >140; R >30, <10; T >38.5°C; pulse oximeter <90%
5. **Activity:** Up as tolerated.
6. **Nursing:** Pulse oximeter, bedside peak flow rate before and after bronchodilator treatments.
7. **Diet:** Regular, no caffeine.
8. **IV Fluids:** D5 ½ NS at 125 cc/h.
9. **Special Medications:**
   -Oxygen 2 L/min by NC. Keep O_2 sat >90%.

Beta Agonists, Acute Treatment:
   -Albuterol (Ventolin) 0.5 mg and ipratropium (Atrovent) 0.5 mg in 2.5 mL NS q1-2h until peak flow meter ≥200-250 L/min and sat ≥90%, then q4h **OR**
   -Albuterol (Ventolin) MDI 3-8 puffs, then 2 puffs q3-6h prn, or powder 200 mcg/capsule inhaled qid.
   -Albuterol/Ipratropium (Combivent) 2-4 puffs qid.

Systemic Corticosteroids:
   -Methylprednisolone (Solu-Medrol) 60-125 mg IV q6h; then 30-60 mg PO qd. **OR**
   -Prednisone 20-60 mg PO qAM.

Aminophylline and Theophylline (second-line therapy):
   -Aminophylline load dose: 5.6 mg/kg **total** body weight in 100 mL D5W IV over 20min. Maintenance of 0.5-0.6 mg/kg **ideal** body weight/h (500 mg in 250 mL D5W); reduce if elderly, heart/liver failure (0.2-0.4 mg/kg/hr). Reduce load 50-75% if taking theophylline (1 mg/kg of aminophylline will raise levels 2 mcg/mL) **OR**
   -Theophylline IV solution loading dose 4.5 mg/kg **total** body weight, then 0.4-0.5 mg/kg **ideal** body weight/hr.
   -Theophylline (Theo-Dur) 100-400 mg PO bid (3 mg/kg q8h); 80% of total daily IV aminophylline in 2-3 doses.

Inhaled Corticosteroids (adjunct therapy):
   -Beclomethasone (Beclovent) MDI 4-8 puffs bid, with spacer 5 min after bronchodilator, followed by gargling with water
   -Triamcinolone (Azmacort) MDI 2 puffs tid-qid or 4 puffs bid.
   -Flunisolide (AeroBid) MDI 2-4 puffs bid.
   -Fluticasone (Flovent) 2-4 puffs bid (44 or 110 mcg/puff); requires 1-2 weeks for full effect.

Maintenance Treatment:
   -Salmeterol (Serevent) 2 puffs bid; not effective for acute asthma because of delayed onset of action.
   -Pirbuterol (Maxair) MDI 2 puffs q4-6h prn.
   -Bitolterol (Tornalate) MDI 2-3 puffs q1-3min, then 2-3 puffs q4-8h prn.
   -Fenoterol (Berotec) MDI 3 puffs, then 2 bid-qid.
   -Ipratropium (Atrovent) MDI 2-3 puffs tid-qid.

Prevention and Prophylaxis:
-Cromolyn (Intal) 2-4 puffs tid-qid.
-Nedocromil (Tilade) 2-4 puffs bid-qid.
-Montelukast (Singulair) 10 mg PO qd.
-Zafirlukast (Accolate) 20 mg PO bid.
-Zileuton (Zyflo) 600 mg PO qid.

Acute Bronchitis
-Ampicillin/sulbactam (Unasyn) 1.5 gm IV q6h **OR**
-Cefuroxime (Zinacef) 750 mg IV q8h **OR**
-Cefuroxime axetil (Ceftin) 250-500 mg PO bid **OR**
-Trimethoprim/sulfamethoxazole (Bactrim DS), 1 tab PO bid **OR**
-Levofloxacin (Levaquin) 500 mg PO/IV PO qd [250, 500 mg].
-Amoxicillin 875 mg/clavulanate 125 mg (Augmentin 875) 1 tab PO bid.

10. Symptomatic Medications:
-Docusate sodium (Colace) 100 mg PO qhs.
-Famotidine (Pepcid) 20 mg IV/PO q12h.
-Acetaminophen (Tylenol) 325-650 mg PO q4-6h prn headache.
-Zolpidem (Ambien) 5-10 mg qhs prn insomnia.

11. Extras: Portable CXR, ECG, pulmonary function tests before and after bronchodilators; pulmonary rehabilitation; impedance cardiography, echocardiogram.

12. Labs: ABG, CBC with eosinophil count, SMA7, B-type natriuretic peptide (BNP). Theophylline level stat and after 24h of infusion. Sputum Gram stain, C&S.

Chronic Obstructive Pulmonary Disease

1. Admit to:
2. Diagnosis: Exacerbation of COPD
3. Condition:
4. Vital Signs: q4h. Call physician if P >130; R >30, <10; T >38.5°C; O_2 Sat <90%.
5. Activity: Up as tolerated; bedside commode.
6. Nursing: Pulse oximeter. Measure peak flow with portable peak flow meter bid and chart with vital signs. No sedatives.
7. Diet: No added salt, no caffeine. Push fluids.
8. IV Fluids: D5 ½ NS with 20 mEq KCL/L at 125 cc/h.
9. Special Medications:
-Oxygen 1-2 L/min by NC or 24-35% by Venturi mask, keep O_2 saturation 90-91%.

Beta-Agonists, Acute Treatment:
-Albuterol (Ventolin) 0.5 mg and ipratropium (Atrovent) 0.5 mg in 2.5 mL NS q1-2h until peak flow meter ≥200-250 L/min, then q4h **OR**
-Albuterol (Ventolin) MDI 2-4 puffs q4-6h.
-Albuterol/Ipratropium (Combivent) 2-4 puffs qid.

Corticosteroids and Anticholinergics:
-Methylprednisolone (Solu-Medrol) 60-125 mg IV q6h or 30-60 mg PO qd.
   Followed by:
-Prednisone 20-60 mg PO qd.
-Triamcinolone (Azmacort) MDI 2 puffs qid or 4 puffs bid.
-Beclomethasone (Beclovent) MDI 4-8 puffs bid with spacer, followed by gar-

gling with water **OR**
-Flunisolide (AeroBid) MDI 2-4 puffs bid **OR**
-Ipratropium (Atrovent) MDI 2 puffs tid-qid **OR**
-Fluticasone (Flovent) 2-4 puffs bid (44 or 110 mcg/puff).

Aminophylline and Theophylline (second line therapy):
-Aminophylline loading dose, 5.6 mg/kg **total** body weight over 20 min (if not already on theophylline); then 0.5-0.6 mg/kg **ideal** body weight/hr (500 mg in 250 mL of D5W); reduce if elderly, or heart or liver disease (0.2-0.4 mg/kg/hr). Reduce loading to 50-75% if already taking theophylline (1 mg/kg of aminophylline will raise levels by 2 mcg/mL) **OR**
-Theophylline IV solution loading dose, 4.5 mg/kg **total** body weight, then 0.4-0.5 mg/kg **ideal** body weight/hr.
-Theophylline long acting (Theo-Dur) 100-400 mg PO bid-tid (3 mg/kg q8h); 80% of daily IV aminophylline in 2-3 doses.

Acute Bronchitis
-Ampicillin 1 gm IV q6h or 500 mg PO qid **OR**
-Trimethoprim/sulfamethoxazole (Septra DS) 160/800 mg PO bid or 160/800 mg IV q12h (10-15 mL in 100 cc D5W tid) **OR**
-Cefuroxime (Zinacef) 750 mg IV q8h **OR**
-Ampicillin/sulbactam (Unasyn) 1.5 gm IV q6h **OR**
-Doxycycline (Vibra-tabs) 100 mg PO/IV bid
-Azithromycin (Zithromax) 500 mg x 1, then 250 mg PO qd x 4 or 500 mg IV q24h **OR**
-Clarithromycin (Biaxin) 250-500 mg PO bid **OR**
-Levofloxacin (Levaquin) 500 mg PO/IV qd [250, 500 mg] **OR**
-Sparfloxacin (Zagam) 400 mg PO x 1, then 200 mg PO qd [200 mg].

10. Symptomatic Medications:
-Docusate sodium (Colace) 100 mg PO qhs.
-Famotidine (Pepcid) 20 mg IV/PO q12h.
-Acetaminophen (Tylenol) 325-650 mg PO q4-6h prn headache.
-Zolpidem (Ambien) 5-10 mg qhs prn insomnia.

11. Extras: Portable CXR, PFT's with bronchodilators, ECG, impedance cardiography, echocardiogram.

12. Labs: ABG, CBC, SMA7, UA. Theophylline level stat and after 12-24h of infusion. Sputum Gram stain and C&S, alpha 1 antitrypsin level.

Hemoptysis

1. Admit to: Intensive care unit
2. Diagnosis: Hemoptysis
3. Condition:
4. Vital Signs: q1-6h. Orthostatic BP and pulse bid. Call physician if BP >160/90, <90/60; P >130, <50; R>25, <10; T >38.5°C; O_2 sat <90%.
5. Activity: Bed rest with bedside commode. Keep patient in lateral decubitus, Trendelenburg's position, bleeding side down.
6. Nursing: Quantify all sputum and expectorated blood, suction prn. O_2 at 100% by mask, pulse oximeter. Discontinue narcotics and sedatives. Have double lumen endotracheal tube available for use.
7. Diet:
8. IV Fluids: 1 L of NS wide open (≥6 gauge), then transfuse PRBC, Foley to gravity.

9. **Special Medications:**
   -Transfuse 2-4 U PRBC wide open.
   -Promethazine/codeine (Phenergan with codeine) 5 cc PO q4-6h prn cough. Contraindicated in massive hemoptysis.
   -Initiate empiric antibiotics if bronchitis or infection is present.
10. **Extras:** CXR PA, LAT, ECG, VQ scan, contrast CT, bronchoscopy. PPD, pulmonary and thoracic surgery consults.
11. **Labs:** Type and cross 2-4 U PRBC. ABG, CBC, platelets, SMA7 and 12, ESR. Anti-glomerular basement antibody, rheumatoid factor, complement, anti-nuclear cytoplasmic antibody. Sputum Gram stain, C&S, AFB, fungal culture, and cytology qAM for 3 days. UA, INR/PTT, von Willebrand Factor. Repeat CBC q6h.

Anaphylaxis

1. **Admit to:**
2. **Diagnosis:** Anaphylaxis
3. **Condition:**
4. **Vital Signs:** q1-4h; call physician if BP systolic >160, <90; diastolic >90, <60; P >120, <50; R>25, <10; T >38.5°C
5. **Activity:** Bedrest
6. **Nursing:** O_2 at 6 L/min by NC or mask. Keep patient in Trendelenburg's position, No. 4 or 5 endotracheal tube at bedside.
7. **Diet:** NPO
8. **IV Fluids:** 2 IV lines. Normal saline or LR 1 L over 1-2h, then D5 ½ NS at 125 cc/h. Foley to closed drainage.
9. **Special Medications:**

Gastrointestinal Decontamination:
   -Gastric lavage if indicated for recent oral ingestion.
   -Activated charcoal 50-100 gm, followed by cathartic.

Bronchodilators:
   -Epinephrine (1:1000) 0.3-0.5 mL SQ or IM q10min or 1-4 mcg/min IV **OR** in severe life threatening reactions, give 0.5 mg (5.0 mL of 1: 10,000 sln) IV q5-10min prn. Epinephrine, 0.3 mg of 1:1000 sln may be injected SQ at site of allergen injection **OR**
   -Albuterol (Ventolin) 0.5%, 0.5 mL in 2.5 mL NS q30min by nebulizer prn **OR**
   -Aerosolized 2% racemic epinephrine 0.5-0.75 mL.

Corticosteroids:
   -Methylprednisolone (Solu-Medrol) 250 mg IV x 1, then 125 mg IV q6h **OR**
   -Hydrocortisone sodium succinate 200 mg IV x 1, then 100 mg q6h, followed by oral prednisone 60 mg PO qd, tapered over 5 days.

Antihistamines:
   -Diphenhydramine (Benadryl) 25-50 mg IV q4-6h **OR**
   -Hydroxyzine (Vistaril) 25-50 mg IM or PO q2-4h.
   -Famotidine (Pepcid) 20 mg IV/PO bid.

Pressors and other Agents:
   -Norepinephrine (Levophed) 8-12 mcg/min IV, titrate to systolic 100 mmHg (8 mg in 500 mL D5W) **OR**
   -Dopamine (Intropin) 5-20 mcg/kg/min IV.
10. **Extras:** Portable CXR, ECG, allergy consult.
11. **Labs:** CBC, SMA 7&12.

Pleural Effusion

1. **Admit to:**
2. **Diagnosis:** Pleural effusion
3. **Condition:**
4. **Vital Signs:** q shift. Call physician if BP >160/90, <90/60; P>120, <50; R>25, <10; T >38.5°C
5. **Activity:**
6. **Diet:** Regular.
7. **IV Fluids:** D5W at TKO
8. **Extras:** CXR PA and LAT, repeat after thoracentesis; left and right lateral decubitus x-rays, ECG, ultrasound, PPD; pulmonary consult.
9. **Labs:** CBC, SMA 7&12, protein, albumin, amylase, ANA, ESR, INR/PTT, UA. Cryptococcal antigen, histoplasma antigen, fungal culture.

Thoracentesis:

Tube 1: LDH, protein, amylase, triglyceride, glucose (10 mL).

Tube 2: Gram stain, C&S, AFB, fungal C&S (20-60 mL, heparinized).

Tube 3: Cell count and differential (5-10 mL, EDTA).

Syringe: pH (2 mL collected anaerobically, heparinized on ice).

Bag or Bottle: Cytology.

38 Pleural Effusion

Hematologic Disorders

Anticoagulant Overdose

Unfractionated Heparin Overdose:
1. Discontinue heparin infusion.
2. Protamine sulfate, 1 mg IV for every 100 units of heparin infused in preceding hour, dilute in 25 mL fluid IV over 10 min (max 50 mg in 10 min period).

Low Molecular Weight Heparin (Enoxaparin) Overdose:
-Protamine sulfate 1 mg IV for each 1 mg of enoxaparin given. Repeat protamine 0.5 mg IV for each 1 mg of enoxaparin, if bleeding continues after 2-4 hours. Measure factor Xa.

Warfarin (Coumadin) Overdose:
-Gastric lavage and activated charcoal if recent oral ingestion. Discontinue Coumadin and heparin, and monitor hematocrit q2h.

Partial Reversal:
-Vitamin K (Phytonadione), 0.5-1.0 mg IV/SQ. Check INR in 24 hours, and repeat vitamin K dose if INR remains elevated.

Minor Bleeds:
-Vitamin K (Phytonadione), 5-10 mg IV/SQ q12h, titrated to desired INR.

Serious Bleeds:
-Vitamin K (Phytonadione), 10-20 mg in 50-100 mL fluid IV over 30-60 min (check INR q6h until corrected) **AND**
-Fresh frozen plasma 2-4 units x 1.
-Type and cross match for 2 units of PRBC, and transfuse wide open.
-Cryoprecipitate 10 U x 1 if fibrinogen is less than100 mg/dL.

Labs: CBC, platelets, PTT, INR.

Deep Venous Thrombosis

1. **Admit to:**
2. **Diagnosis:** Deep vein thrombosis
3. **Condition:**
4. **Vital Signs:** q shift. Call physician if BP systolic >160, <90 diastolic, >90, <60; P >120, <50; R>25, <10; T >38.5°C.
5. **Activity:** Bed rest with legs elevated.
6. **Nursing:** Guaiac stools, warm packs to leg prn; measure calf and thigh circumference qd; no intramuscular injections.
7. **Diet:** Regular
8. **IV Fluids:** D5W at TKO
9. **Special Medications:**

Anticoagulation:
-Heparin (unfractionated) IV bolus 5000-10,000 Units (100 U/kg) IVP, then 1000-1500 U/h IV infusion (20 U/kg/h) [25,000 U in 500 mL D5W (50 U/mL)]. Check PTT 6 hours after initial bolus; adjust q6h until PTT 1.5-2.0 times control (50-80 sec). Overlap heparin and warfarin (Coumadin) for at least 4 days and discontinue heparin when INR has been 2.0-3.0 for two

    consecutive days.
  -Enoxaparin (Lovenox) 1 mg/kg SQ q12h or 1.5 mg/kg SQ q24 h for DVT
    without pulmonary embolism. Overlap enoxaparin and warfarin as outlined
    above.
  -Warfarin (Coumadin) 5-10 mg PO qd x 2-3 d; maintain INR 2.0-3.0.
    Coumadin is initiated on the first or second day only if the PTT is 1.5-2.0
    times control [tab 1, 2, 2.5, 3, 4, 5, 6, 7.5, 10 mg].
10. Symptomatic Medications:
  -Propoxyphene/acetaminophen (Darvocet N100) 1-2 tab PO q3-4h prn pain
      OR
  -Hydrocodone/acetaminophen (Vicodin), 1-2 tab q4-6h PO prn pain.
  -Docusate sodium (Colace) 100 mg PO qhs.
  -Famotidine (Pepcid) 20 mg IV/PO q12h.
  -Zolpidem (Ambien) 5-10 mg qhs prn insomnia.
11. Extras: CXR PA and LAT, ECG; Doppler scan of legs. V/Q scan, chest CT
    scan.
12. Labs: CBC, INR/PTT, SMA 7. Protein C, protein S, antithrombin III,
    anticardiolipin antibody. UA with dipstick for blood. PTT 6h after bolus and q4-
    6h until PTT 1.5-2.0 x control then qd. INR at initiation of warfarin and qd.

Pulmonary Embolism

1. **Admit to:**
2. **Diagnosis:** Pulmonary embolism
3. **Condition:**
4. **Vital Signs:** q1-4h. Call physician if BP >160/90, <90/60; P >120, <50; R >30,
    <10; T >38.5°C; O₂ sat < 90%
5. **Activity:** Bedrest with bedside commode
6. **Nursing:** Pulse oximeter, guaiac stools, O₂ at 2 L by NC. Antiembolism
    stockings. No intramuscular injections.
7. **Diet:** Regular
8. **IV Fluids:** D5W at TKO.
9. **Special Medications:**
Anticoagulation:
  -Heparin IV bolus 5000-10,000 Units (100 U/kg) IVP, then 1000-1500 U/h IV
    infusion (20 U/kg/h) [25,000 U in 500 mL D5W (50 U/mL)]. Check PTT 6
    hours after initial bolus; adjust q6h until PTT 1.5-2 times control (60-80
    sec). Overlap heparin and Coumadin for at least 4 days and discontinue
    heparin when INR has been 2.0-3.0 for two consecutive days.
  -Enoxaparin (Lovenox) 1 mg/kg sq q12h for 5 days for uncomplicated
    pulmonary embolism. Overlap warfarin as outlined above.
  -Warfarin (Coumadin) 5-10 mg PO qd for 2-3 d, then 2-5 mg PO qd. Maintain
    INR of 2.0-3.0. Coumadin is initiated on second day if the PTT is 1.5-2.0
    times control. Check INR at initiation of warfarin and qd [tab 1, 2, 2.5, 3, 4,
    5, 6, 7.5, 10 mg].
Thrombolytics (indicated if hemodynamic compromise):
  Baseline Labs: CBC, INR/PTT, fibrinogen q6h.
  Alteplase (recombinant tissue plasminogen activator, Activase): 100 mg
    IV infusion over 2 hours, followed by heparin infusion at 15 U/kg/h to
    maintain PTT 1.5-2.5 x control **OR**
  Streptokinase (Streptase): Pretreat with methylprednisolone 250 mg IV

push and diphenhydramine (Benadryl) 50 mg IV push. Then give streptokinase, 250,000 units IV over 30 min, then 100,000 units/h for 24-72 hours. Initiate heparin infusion at 10 U/kg/hour; maintain PTT 1.5-2.5 x control.

10. **Symptomatic Medications:**
-Meperidine (Demerol) 25-100 mg IV prn pain.
-Docusate sodium (Colace) 100 mg PO qhs.
-Famotidine (Pepcid) 20 mg IV/PO q12h.

11. **Extras:** CXR PA and LAT, ECG, VQ scan; chest CT scan, pulmonary angiography; Doppler scan of lower extremities, impedance cardiography.

12. **Labs:** CBC, INR/PTT, SMA7, ABG, cardiac enzymes. Protein C, protein S, antithrombin III, anticardiolipin antibody. UA . PTT 6 hours after bolus and q4-6h. INR at initiation of warfarin and qd.

Sickle Cell Crisis

1. **Admit to:**
2. **Diagnosis:** Sickle Cell Crisis
3. **Condition:**
4. **Vital Signs:** q shift.
5. **Activity:** Bedrest
6. **Nursing:**
7. **Diet:** Regular diet, push oral fluids.
8. **IV Fluids:** D5 ½ NS at 100-125 mL/h.
9. **Special Medications:**
-Oxygen 2 L/min by NC or 30-100% by mask.
-Meperidine (Demerol) 50-150 mg IM/IV q4-6h prn pain.
-Hydroxyzine (Vistaril) 25-100 mg IM/IV/PO q3-4h prn pain.
-Morphine sulfate 10 mg IV/IM/SC q2-4h prn pain **OR**
-Ketorolac (Toradol) 30-60 mg IV/IM then 15-30 mg IV/IM q6h prn pain (maximum of 5 days).
-Acetaminophen/codeine (Tylenol 3) 1-2 tabs PO q4-6h prn.
-Folic acid 1 mg PO qd.
-Penicillin V (prophylaxis), 250 mg PO qid [tabs 125,250,500 mg].
-Ondansetron (Zofran) 4 mg PO/IV q4-6h prn nausea or vomiting.

10. **Symptomatic Medications:**
-Zolpidem (Ambien) 5-10 mg qhs prn insomnia.
-Docusate sodium (Colace) 100-200 mg PO qhs.

Vaccination:
-Pneumovax before discharge 0.5 cc IM x 1 dose.
-Influenza vaccine (Fluogen) 0.5 cc IM once a year in the Fall.

11. **Extras:** CXR.

12. **Labs:** CBC, SMA 7, blood C&S, reticulocyte count, blood type and screen, parvovirus titers. UA.

Infectious Diseases

Meningitis

1. **Admit to:**
2. **Diagnosis:** Meningitis.
3. **Condition:**
4. **Vital Signs:** q1h. Call physician if BP systolic >160/90, <90/60; P >120, <50; R>25, <10; T >39°C or less than 36°C
5. **Activity:** Bed rest with bedside commode.
6. **Nursing:** Respiratory isolation, inputs and outputs, lumbar puncture tray at bedside.
7. **Diet:** NPO
8. **IV Fluids:** D5 ½ NS at 125 cc/h with KCL 20 mEq/L.
9. **Special Medications:**

Empiric Therapy 15-50 years old:
   -Vancomycin 1 gm IV q12h **AND EITHER**
   -Ceftriaxone (Rocephin) 2 gm IV q12h (max 4 gm/d) **OR**
   Cefotaxime (Claforan) 2 gm IV q4h.

Empiric Therapy >50 years old, Alcoholic, Corticosteroids or Hematologic Malignancy or other Debilitating Condition:
   -Ampicillin 2 gm IV q4h **AND EITHER**
   -Cefotaxime (Claforan) 2 gm IV q6h **OR**
   Ceftriaxone (Rocephin) 2 gm IV q12h **OR**
   Ceftazidime (Fortaz) 2 gm IV q8h.
   -Use Vancomycin 1 gm IV q12h in place of ampicillin if drug-resistant pneumococcus is suspected.

10. **Symptomatic Medications:**
    -Heparin 5000 U SC q12h or pneumatic compression stockings.
    -Famotidine (Pepcid) 20 mg IV/PO q12h.
    -Acetaminophen (Tylenol) 650 mg PO/PR q4-6h prn temp >39˚C.
    -Docusate sodium 100-200 mg PO qhs.
11. **Extras:** CXR, ECG, PPD, CT scan.
12. **Labs:** CBC, SMA 7&12. Blood C&S x 2. UA with micro, urine C&S. Antibiotic levels peak and trough after 3rd dose, VDRL.

Lumbar Puncture:
   CSF Tube 1: Gram stain, C&S for bacteria (1-4 mL).
   CSF Tube 2: Glucose, protein (1-2 mL).
   CSF Tube 3: Cell count and differential (1-2 mL).
   CSF Tube 4: Latex agglutination or counterimmunoelectrophoresis antigen tests for S. pneumoniae, H. influenzae (type B), N. meningitides, E. coli, group B strep, VDRL, cryptococcal antigen, toxoplasma titers. India ink, fungal cultures, AFB (8-10 mL).

Infective Endocarditis

1. **Admit to:**
2. **Diagnosis:** Infective endocarditis
3. **Condition:**
4. **Vital Signs:** q4h. Call physician if BP systolic >160/90, <90/60; P >120, <50; R>25, <10; T >38.5°C
5. **Activity:** Up ad lib
6. **Diet:** Regular
7. **IV Fluids:** Heparin lock with flush q shift.
8. **Special Medications:**

Subacute Bacterial Endocarditis Empiric Therapy:
  -Penicillin G 3-5 million U IV q4h or ampicillin 2 gm IV q4h **AND**
  Gentamicin 1-1.5/kg IV q8h.

Acute Bacterial Endocarditis Empiric Therapy
  -Gentamicin 2 mg/kg IV; then 1-1.5 mg/kg IV q8h **AND**
  Nafcillin or oxacillin 2 gm IV q4h **OR**
  Vancomycin 1 gm IV q12h (1 gm in 250 mL of D5W over 1h).

Streptococci viridans/bovis:
  -Penicillin G 3-5 million U IV q4h for 4 weeks **OR**
  Vancomycin 1 gm IV q12h for 4 weeks **AND**
  Gentamicin 1 mg/kg q8h for first 2 weeks.

Enterococcus:
  -Gentamicin 1 mg/kg IV q8h for 4-6 weeks **AND**
  Ampicillin 2 gm IV q4h for 4-6 weeks **OR**
  Vancomycin 1 gm IV q12h for 4-6 weeks.

Staphylococcus aureus (methicillin sensitive, native valve):
  -Nafcillin or Oxacillin 2 gm IV q4h for 4-6 weeks **OR**
  Vancomycin 1 gm IV q12h for 4-6 weeks **AND**
  Gentamicin 1 mg/kg IV q8h for first 3-5 days.

Methicillin resistant Staphylococcus aureus (native valve):
  -Vancomycin 1 gm IV q12h (1 gm in 250 mL D5W over 1h) for 4-6 weeks **AND**
  Gentamicin 1 mg/kg IV q8h for 3-5 days.

Methicillin resistant Staph aureus or epidermidis (prosthetic valve):
  -Vancomycin 1 gm IV q12h for 6 weeks **AND**
  Rifampin 600 mg PO q8h for 6 weeks **AND**
  Gentamicin 1 mg/kg IV q8h for 2 weeks.

Culture Negative Endocarditis:
  -Penicillin G 3-5 million U IV q4h for 4-6 weeks **OR**
  Ampicillin 2 gm IV q4h for 4-6 weeks **AND**
  Gentamicin 1.5 mg/kg q8h for 2 weeks (or nafcillin, 2 gm IV q4h, and gentamicin if Staph aureus suspected in drug abuser or prosthetic valve).

Fungal Endocarditis:
  -Amphotericin B 0.5 mg/kg/d IV plus flucytosine (5-FC) 150 mg/kg/d PO.

9. **Symptomatic Medications:**
  -Acetaminophen (Tylenol) 325-650 mg PO q4-6h prn temp >39° C.
  -Docusate sodium 100-200 mg PO qhs.
10. **Extras:** CXR PA and LAT, echocardiogram, ECG.
11. **Labs:** CBC with differential, SMA 7&12. Blood C&S x 3-4 over 24h, serum cidal titers, minimum inhibitory concentration, minimum bactericidal concentration. Repeat C&S in 48h, then once a week. Antibiotic levels peak

and trough at 3rd dose. UA, urine C&S.

Pneumonia

1. **Admit to:**
2. **Diagnosis:** Pneumonia
3. **Condition:**
4. **Vital Signs:** q4-8h. Call physician if BP >160/90, <90/60; P >120, <50; R>25, <10; T >38.5°C or O_2 saturation <90%.
5. **Activity:**
6. **Nursing:** Pulse oximeter, inputs and outputs, nasotracheal suctioning prn, incentive spirometry.
7. **Diet:** Regular.
8. **IV Fluids:** IV D5 ½ NS at 125 cc/hr.
9. **Special Medications:**
   -Oxygen by NC at 2-4 L/min, or 24-50% by Ventimask, or 100% by non-rebreather (reservoir) to maintain O_2 saturation >90%.

Moderately ill Patients Without Underlying Lung Disease from the Community:
   -Cefuroxime (Zinacef) 0.75-1.5 gm IV q8h **OR**
   Ampicillin/sulbactam (Unasyn) 1.5 gm IV q6h **AND EITHER**
   -Erythromycin 500 mg IV/PO q6h **OR**
   Clarithromycin (Biaxin) 500 mg PO bid **OR**
   Azithromycin (Zithromax) 500 mg PO x 1, then 250 mg PO qd x 4 **OR**
   Doxycycline (Vibramycin) 100 mg IV/PO q12h.

Moderately ill Patients With Recent Hospitalization or Debilitated Nursing Home Patient:
   -Ceftazidime (Fortaz) 1-2 gm IV q8h **OR**
   Cefepime (Maxipime) 1-2 gm IV q12h **AND EITHER**
   Gentamicin 1.5-2 mg/kg IV, then 1.0-1.5 mg/kg IV q8h or 7 mg/kg in 50 mL of D5W over 60 min IV q24h **OR**
   -Ciprofloxacin (Cipro) 400 mg IV q12h or 500 mg PO q12h.

Critically ill Patients:
   -Initial treatment should consist of a macrolide with 2 antipseudomonal agents for synergistic activity:
   -Erythromycin 0.5-1.0 gm IV q6h **AND EITHER**
   -Ceftazidime 1-2 gm q8h **OR**
   Piperacillin/tazobactam (Zosyn) 3.75-4.50 gm IV q6h **OR**
   Ticarcillin/clavulanate (Timentin) 3.1 gm IV q6h **OR**
   Imipenem/cilastatin (Primaxin) 0.5-1.0 gm IV q6h **AND EITHER**
   -Levofloxacin (Levaquin) 500 mg IV q24h **OR**
   Ciprofloxacin (Cipro) 400 mg IV q12h **OR**
   Tobramycin 2.0 mg/kg IV, then 1.5 mg/kg IV q8h or 7 mg/kg IV q24h.

Aspiration Pneumonia (community acquired):
   -Clindamycin (Cleocin) 600-900 mg IV q8h (with or without gentamicin or 3rd gen cephalosporin) **OR**
   -Ampicillin/sulbactam (Unasyn) 1.5-3 gm IV q6h (with or without gentamicin or 3rd gen cephalosporin)

Aspiration Pneumonia (nosocomial):
   -Tobramycin 2 mg/kg IV then 1.5 mg/kg IV q8h or 7 mg/kg in 50 mL of D5W over 60 min IV q24h **OR**

Ceftazidime (Fortaz) 1-2 gm IV q8h **AND EITHER**
-Clindamycin (Cleocin) 600-900 mg IV q8h **OR**
Ampicillin/sulbactam or ticarcillin/clavulanate, or piperacillin/tazobactam or
    imipenem/cilastatin (see above) **OR**
Metronidazole (Flagyl) 500 mg IV q8h.

10. Symptomatic Medications:
-Acetaminophen (Tylenol) 650 mg 2 tab PO q4-6h prn temp >38°C or pain.
-Docusate sodium (Colace) 100 mg PO qhs.
-Famotidine (Pepcid) 20 mg IV/PO q12h.
-Heparin 5000 U SQ q12h or pneumatic compression stockings.

11. Extras: CXR PA and LAT, ECG, PPD.

12. Labs: CBC with differential, SMA 7&12, ABG. Blood C&S x 2. Sputum Gram
stain, C&S. Methenamine silver sputum stain (PCP); AFB smear/culture.
Aminoglycoside levels peak and trough at 3rd dose. UA, urine culture.

Specific Therapy for Pneumonia

Pneumococcus:
-Ceftriaxone (Rocephin) 2 gm IV q12h **OR**
-Cefotaxime (Claforan) 2 gm IV q6h **OR**
-Erythromycin 500 mg IV q6h **OR**
-Vancomycin 1 gm IV q12h if drug resistance.

Staphylococcus aureus:
-Nafcillin 2 gm IV q4h **OR**
-Oxacillin 2 gm IV q4h.

Klebsiella pneumoniae:
-Gentamicin 1.5-2 mg/kg IV, then 1.0-1.5 mg/kg IV q8h or 7 mg/kg in 50 mL
    of D5W over 60 min IV q24h **OR**
Ceftizoxime (Cefizox) 1-2 gm IV q8h **OR**
Cefotaxime (Claforan) 1-2 gm IV q6h.

Methicillin-resistant staphylococcus aureus (MRSA):
-Vancomycin 1 gm IV q12h.

Vancomycin-Resistant Enterococcus:
-Linezolid (Zyvox) 600 mg IV/PO q12h; active against MRSA as well **OR**
-Quinupristin/dalfopristin (Synercid) 7.5 mg/kg IV q8h; does not cover E
    faecalis.

Haemophilus influenzae:
-Ampicillin 1-2 gm IV q6h (beta-lactamase negative) **OR**
-Ampicillin/sulbactam (Unasyn) 1.5-3.0 gm q6h **OR**
-Cefuroxime (Zinacef) 1.5 gm IV q8h (beta-lactamase pos) **OR**
-Ceftizoxime (Cefizox) 1-2 gm IV q8h **OR**
-Ciprofloxacin (Cipro) 400 mg IV q12h **OR**
-Ofloxacin (Floxin) 400 mg IV q12h.
-Levofloxacin (Levaquin) 500 mg IV q24h.

Pseudomonas aeruginosa:
-Tobramycin 1.5-2.0 mg/kg IV, then 1.5-2.0 mg/kg IV q8h or 7 mg/kg in 50 mL
    of D5W over 60 min IV q24h **AND EITHER**
Piperacillin, Ticarcillin, Mezlocillin or Azlocillin 3 gm IV q4h **OR**
Ceftazidime 1-2 gm IV q8h.

Enterobacter Aerogenes or Cloacae:
-Gentamicin 2.0 mg/kg IV, then 1.5 mg/kg IV q8h **AND EITHER**

Meropenem (Merrem) 1 gm IV q8h **OR**
Imipenem/cilastatin (Primaxin) 0.5-1.0 gm IV q6h.

Serratia Marcescens:
-Ceftizoxime (Cefizox) 1-2 gm IV q8h **OR**
-Aztreonam (Azactam) 1-2 gm IV q6h **OR**
-Imipenem/cilastatin (Primaxin) 0.5-1.0 gm IV q6h **OR**
-Meropenem (Merrem) 1 gm IV q8h.

Mycoplasma pneumoniae:
-Clarithromycin (Biaxin) 500 mg PO bid **OR**
-Azithromycin (Zithromax) 500 mg PO x 1, then 250 mg PO qd for 4 days **OR**
-Erythromycin 500 mg PO or IV q6h **OR**
-Doxycycline (Vibramycin) 100 mg PO/IV q12h **OR**
-Levofloxacin (Levaquin) 500 mg PO/IV q24h.

Legionella pneumoniae:
-Erythromycin 1.0 gm IV q6h **OR**
-Levofloxacin (Levaquin) 500 mg PO/IV q24h.
-Rifampin 600 mg PO qd may be added to erythromycin or levofloxacin.

Moraxella catarrhalis:
-Trimethoprim/sulfamethoxazole (Bactrim, Septra) one DS tab PO bid or 10 mL IV q12h **OR**
-Ampicillin/sulbactam (Unasyn) 1.5-3 gm IV q6h **OR**
-Cefuroxime (Zinacef) 0.75-1.5 gm IV q8h **OR**
-Erythromycin 500 mg IV q6h **OR**
-Levofloxacin (Levaquin) 500 mg PO/IV q24h.

Anaerobic Pneumonia:
-Penicillin G 2 MU IV q4h **OR**
-Clindamycin (Cleocin) 900 mg IV q8h **OR**
-Metronidazole (Flagyl) 500 mg IV q8h.

Pneumocystis Carinii Pneumonia and HIV

1. **Admit to:**
2. **Diagnosis:** PCP pneumonia
3. **Condition:**
4. **Vital Signs:** q2-6h. Call physician if BP >160/90, <90/60; P >120, <50; R>25, <10; T >38.5°C; O_2 sat <90%
5. **Activity:**
6. **Nursing:** Pulse oximeter.
7. **Diet:** Regular, encourage fluids.
8. **IV Fluids:** D5 ½ NS at 100 cc/h.
9. **Special Medications:**

Pneumocystis Carinii Pneumonia:
-Oxygen at 2-4 L/min by NC or by mask.
-Trimethoprim/sulfamethoxazole (Bactrim, Septra) 15 mg of TMP/kg/day (20 mL in 250 mL of D5W IVPB q8h) for 21 days [inj: 80/400 mg per 5 mL].
-If severe PCP (PaO_2 <70 mmHg): add prednisone 40 mg PO bid for 5 days, then 40 mg qd for 5 days, then 20 mg once daily for 11 days **OR** Methylprednisolone (Solu-Medrol) 30 mg IV q12h for 5 days, then 30 mg IV qd for 5 days, then 15 mg IV qd for 11 days.
-Pentamidine (Pentam) 4 mg/kg IV qd for 21 days, with prednisone as above. Pentamidine is an alternative if inadequate response or intolerant to TMP-

SMX.

Pneumocystis Carinii Prophylaxis (previous PCP or CD4 <200, or constitutional symptoms):

-Trimethoprim/SMX DS (160/800 mg) PO qd **OR**

-Pentamidine, 300 mg in 6 mL sterile water via Respirgard II nebulizer over 20-30 min q4 weeks **OR**

-Dapsone (DDS) 50 mg PO bid or 100 mg twice a week; contraindicated in G-6-PD deficiency.

Antiretroviral Therapy:

A. Combination therapy with 3 agents (two nucleoside analogs and a protease inhibitor) is recommended as initial therapy. Nucleotide analogs are similar to nucleosides and may be used interchangeably.

B. Nucleoside Analogs
1. Abacavir (Ziagen) 300 mg PO bid [300 mg, 20 mg/mL].
2. Didanosine (Videx, ddI) 200 mg bid for patients >60 kg; or 125 mg bid for patients <60 kg.[chewable tabs: 25, 50, 100, 150 mg; pwd 100, 167, 250 mg packets].
3. Lamivudine (Epivir, 3TC) 150 mg twice daily [150 mg].
4. Stavudine (Zerit, D4T) 40 mg bid [15-mg, 20-mg, 30-mg and 40-mg capsules].
5. Zalcitabine (Hivid, ddC) 0.75 mg tid [0.375, 0.75].
6. Zidovudine (Retrovir, AZT) 200 mg tid (100, 200 mg caps, 50 mg/5 mL syrup).

C. Protease Inhibitors
1. Amprenavir (Agenerase) 1200 mg bid [50, 150 mg].
2. Indinavir (Crixivan) 800 mg tid [200, 400 mg].
3. Lopinavir/ritonavir (Kaletra) 400 mg/100 mg PO bid.
4. Nelfinavir (Viracept) 750 mg PO tid [250 mg].
5. Ritonavir (Norvir) 600 mg bid [100 mg, 80 mg/dL].
6. Saquinavir (Invirase) 600 mg tid with a meal [cap 200 mg].

D. Non-Nucleoside Reverse Transcriptase Inhibitors
1. Delavirdine (U-90) 400 mg tid.
2. Efavirenz (Sustiva) 600 mg PO qd [50, 100, 200 mg].
3. Nevirapine (Viramune) 200 mg qd for 2 weeks, then bid [200 mg].

E. Nucleotide Analogs
1. Tenofovir (Viread) 300 mg PO qd with food.

Postexposure HIV Prophylaxis

A. The injury should be immediately washed and scrubbed with soap and water.

B. Zidovudine 200 mg PO tid and lamivudine (3TC) 150 mg PO bid, plus indinavir (Crixivan) 800 mg PO tid for highest risk exposures. Treatment is continued for one month.

Zidovudine-Induced Neutropenia/Ganciclovir-Induced Leucopenia

-Recombinant human granulocyte colony-stimulating factor (G-CSF, Filgrastim, Neupogen) 1-2 mcg/kg SQ qd until absolute neutrophil count 500-1000; indicated only if the patient's endogenous erythropoietin level is low.

10. Symptomatic Medications:

-Acetaminophen (Tylenol) 325-650 mg PO q4-6h prn headache.

-Docusate sodium 100-200 mg PO qhs.

10. Extras: CXR PA and LAT.

11. Labs: ABG, CBC, SMA 7&12. Blood C&S x 2. Sputum for Gram stain, C&S, AFB. Giemsa immunofluorescence for Pneumocystis. CD4 count, HIV RNA,

VDRL, serum cryptococcal antigen, UA.

Opportunistic Infections in HIV-Infected Patients

Oral Candidiasis:
- Fluconazole (Diflucan) acute: 100-200 mg PO qd **OR**
- Ketoconazole (Nizoral), acute: 400 mg PO qd **OR**
- Itraconazole (Sporanox) 200 mg PO qd **OR**
- Clotrimazole (Mycelex) troches 10 mg dissolved slowly in mouth 5 times/d.

Candida Esophagitis:
- Fluconazole (Diflucan) 200-400 mg PO qd for 14-21 days **OR**
- Ketoconazole (Nizoral) 200 mg PO bid.
- Itraconazole (Sporanox) 200 mg PO qd for 2 weeks.

Primary or Recurrent Mucocutaneous HSV
- Acyclovir (Zovirax), 200-400 mg PO 5 times a day for 10 days, or 5 mg/kg IV q8h **OR** in cases of acyclovir resistance, foscarnet, 40 mg/kg IV q8h for 21 days.

Herpes Simplex Encephalitis (or visceral disease):
- Acyclovir (Zovirax) 10 mg/kg IV q8h for 10-21 days.

Herpes Varicella Zoster
- Acyclovir (Zovirax) 10 mg/kg IV over 60 min q8h for 7-14 days **OR** 800 mg PO 5 times/d for 7-10 days **OR**
- Famciclovir (Famvir) 500 mg PO q8h for 7 days [500 mg] **OR**
- Valacyclovir (Valtrex) 1000 mg PO q8h for 7 days [500 mg] **OR**
- Foscarnet (Foscavir) 40 mg/kg IV q8h.

Cytomegalovirus Retinitis:
- Ganciclovir (Cytovene) 5 mg/kg IV (dilute in 100 mL D5W over 60 min) q12h for 14-21 days **OR**
- Foscarnet (Foscavir) 60 mg/kg IV q8h for 2-3 weeks **OR**
- Cidofovir (Vistide) 5 mg/kg IV over 60 min q week for 2 weeks. Administer probenecid, 2 g PO 3 hours prior to cidofovir, 1 g PO 2 hours after, and 1 g PO 8 hours after.

Suppressive Treatment for Cytomegalovirus Retinitis:
- Ganciclovir (Cytovene) 5 mg/kg qd.
- Foscarnet (Foscavir) 90-120 mg IV qd **OR**
- Cidofovir (Vistide) 5 mg/kg IV over 60 min every 2 weeks with probenecid.

Acute Toxoplasmosis:
- Pyrimethamine 200 mg, then 50-75 mg qd, plus sulfadiazine 1.0-1.5 gm PO q6h, plus folinic acid 10 mg PO qd **OR**
- Atovaquone (Mepron) 750 mg PO tid.

  Suppressive Treatment for Toxoplasmosis:
  - Pyrimethamine 25-50 mg PO qd plus sulfadiazine 0.5-1.0 gm PO q6h plus folinic acid 5 mg PO qd **OR**
  - Pyrimethamine 50 mg PO qd, plus clindamycin 300 mg PO qid, plus folinic acid 5 mg PO qd.

Cryptococcus Neoformans Meningitis:
- Amphotericin B 0.7-1.0 mg/kg/d IV; total dosage of 2 g, with or without 5-flucytosine 100 mg/kg PO qd in divided doses, followed by fluconazole (Diflucan) 400 mg PO qd or itraconazole (Sporanox) 200 mg PO bid 6-8 weeks
  OR

-Amphotericin B liposomal (Abelcet) 5 mg/kg IV q24h **OR**
-Fluconazole (Diflucan) 400-800 mg PO qd for 8-12 weeks
Suppressive Treatment of Cryptococcus:
   -Fluconazole (Diflucan) 200 mg PO qd indefinitely.
Active Tuberculosis:
   -Isoniazid (INH) 300 mg PO qd; and rifampin 600 mg PO qd; and
      pyrazinamide 15-25 mg/kg PO qd (500 mg bid-tid); and ethambutol 15-25
      mg/kg PO qd (400 mg bid-tid).
   -All four drugs are continued for 2 months; isoniazid and rifampin are
      continued for a period of at least 9 months and at least 6 months after the
      last negative cultures.
   -Pyridoxine (Vitamin B6) 50 mg PO qd concurrent with INH.
Prophylaxis for Inactive Tuberculosis:
   -Isoniazid 300 mg PO qd; and pyridoxine 50 mg PO qd for 12 months.
Disseminated Mycobacterium Avium Complex (MAC):
   -Clarithromycin (Biaxin) 500 mg PO bid **AND**
   Ethambutol 800-1000 mg qd; with or without rifabutin 450 mg qd.
Prophylaxis against Mycobacterium Avium Complex:
   -Azithromycin (Zithromax) 1200 mg once a week.
Disseminated Coccidioidomycosis:
   -Amphotericin (Fungizone) B 0.5-0.8 mg/kg IV qd, to a total dose 2.0 gm **OR**
   -Amphotericin B liposomal (Abelcet) 5 mg/kg IV q24h **OR**
   -Fluconazole (Diflucan) 400-800 mg PO or IV qd.
Disseminated Histoplasmosis:
   -Amphotericin B (Fungizone) 0.5-0.8 mg/kg IV qd, to a total dose 15 mg/kg
      OR
   -Amphotericin B liposomal (Abelcet) 5 mg/kg IV q24h **OR**
   -Fluconazole (Diflucan) 400 mg PO qd. **OR**
   -Itraconazole (Sporanox) 300 mg PO bid for 3 days, then 200 mg PO bid.
Suppressive Treatment for Histoplasmosis:
   -Fluconazole (Diflucan) 400 mg PO qd **OR**
   -Itraconazole (Sporanox) 200 mg PO bid.

Septic Arthritis

1. **Admit to:**
2. **Diagnosis:** Septic arthritis
3. **Condition:**
4. **Vital Signs:** q shift
5. **Activity:** Up in chair as tolerated. Bedside commode with assistance.
6. **Nursing:** Warm compresses prn, keep joint immobilized. Passive range of
   motion exercises of the affected joint bid.
7. **Diet:** Regular diet.
8. **IV Fluids:** Heparin lock
9. **Special Medications:**
Empiric Therapy for Adults without Gonorrhea Contact:
   -Nafcillin or oxacillin 2 gm IV q4h **AND**
   Ceftizoxime (Cefizox) 1 gm IV q8h or ceftazidime 1 gm IV q8h or
   ciprofloxacin 400 mg IV q12h if Gram stain indicates presence of Gram
   negative organisms.

Empiric Therapy for Adults with Gonorrhea:
-Ceftriaxone (Rocephin) 1 gm IV q12h **OR**
-Ceftizoxime (Cefizox) 1 gm IV q8h **OR**
-Ciprofloxacin (Cipro) 400 mg IV q12h.
-Complete course of therapy with cefuroxime axetil (Ceftin) 400 mg PO bid.
10. Symptomatic Medications:
-Acetaminophen and codeine (Tylenol 3) 1-2 PO q4-6h prn pain.
-Heparin 5000 U SQ bid.
-Famotidine (Pepcid) 20 mg IV/PO q12h.
-Zolpidem (Ambien) 5-10 mg qhs prn insomnia.
-Docusate sodium 100-200 mg PO qhs.
11. Extras: X-ray views of joint (AP and lateral), CXR. Synovial fluid culture. Physical therapy consult for exercise program.
12. Labs: CBC, SMA 7&12, blood C&S x 2, VDRL, UA. Gonorrhea cultures of urethra, cervix, urine, throat, sputum, skin, rectum. Antibiotic levels. Blood cultures x 2 for gonorrhea.
Synovial fluid:
Tube 1 - Glucose, protein, lactate, pH.
Tube 2 - Gram stain, C&S.
Tube 3 - Cell count.

Septic Shock

1. Admit to:
2. Diagnosis: Sepsis
3. Condition:
4. Vital Signs: q1h; Call physician if BP >160/90, <90/60; P >120, <50; R>25, <10; T >38.5°C; urine output < 25 cc/hr for 4h, O_2 saturation <90%.
5. Activity: Bed rest.
6. Nursing: Inputs and outputs, pulse oximeter. Foley catheter to closed drainage.
7. Diet: NPO
8. IV Fluids: 1 liter of normal saline wide open, then D5 ½ NS at 125 cc/h
9. Special Medications:
-Oxygen at 2-5 L/min by NC or mask.
Antibiotic Therapy
A. Initial treatment of life-threatening sepsis should include a third-generation cephalosporin (ceftazidime, cefotaxime, ceftizoxime or ceftriaxone), or piperacillin/tazobactam, or ticarcillin/clavulanic acid or imipenem, each with an aminoglycoside (gentamicin, tobramycin or amikacin). If Enterobacter aerogenes or cloacae is suspected, treatment should begin with meropenem, or imipenem with an aminoglycoside.
B. **Intra-abdominal or pelvic infections,** likely to involve anaerobes, should be treated with ampicillin, gentamicin and metronidazole; or either ticarcillin/clavulanic acid, ampicillin/sulbactam, piperacillin/tazobactam, imipenem, cefoxitin or cefotetan, each with an aminoglycoside.
C. **Febrile neutropenic patients** with neutrophil counts <500/mm^3 should be treated with vancomycin and ceftazidime, or piperacillin/tazobactam and tobramycin or imipenem and tobramycin.
D. **Dosages for Antibiotics Used in Sepsis**
-Ampicillin 1-2 gm IV q4h.

-Cefotaxime (Claforan) 2 gm q4-6h.
-Ceftizoxime (Cefizox) 1-2 gm IV q8h.
-Ceftriaxone (Rocephin) 1-2 gm IV q12h (max 4 gm/d).
-Cefoxitin (Mefoxin) 1-2 gm q6h.
-Cefotetan (Cefotan) 1-2 gm IV q12h.
-Ceftazidime (Fortaz) 1-2 g IV q8h.
-Ticarcillin/clavulanate (Timentin) 3.1 gm IV q4-6h (200-300 mg/kg/d).
-Ampicillin/sulbactam (Unasyn) 1.5-3.0 gm IV q6h.
-Piperacillin/tazobactam (Zosyn) 3.375-4.5 gm IV q6h.
-Piperacillin or ticarcillin 3 gm IV q4-6h.
-Imipenem/cilastatin (Primaxin) 1.0 gm IV q6h.
-Meropenem (Merrem) 05-1.0 gm IV q8h.
-Gentamicin, tobramycin 100-120 mg (1.5 mg/kg) IV, then 80 mg IV q8h
  (1 mg/kg) or 7 mg/kg in 50 mL of D5W over 60 min IV q24h.
-Amikacin (Amikin) 7.5 mg/kg IV loading dose; then 5 mg/kg IV q8h.
-Vancomycin 1 gm IV q12h.
-Metronidazole (Flagyl) 500 mg (7.5 mg/kg) IV q6-8h.
-Clindamycin (Cleocin) 900 mg IV q8h.
-Aztreonam (Azactam) 1-2 gm IV q6-8h; max 8 g/day.

Nosocomial sepsis with IV catheter or IV drug abuse
-Nafcillin or oxacillin 2 gm IV q4h **OR**
-Vancomycin 1 gm q12h (1 gm in 250 cc D5W over 60 min) **AND**
 Gentamicin or tobramycin as above **AND EITHER**
 Ceftazidime (Fortaz) or ceftizoxime 1-2 gm IV q8h **OR**
 Piperacillin, ticarcillin or mezlocillin 3 gm IV q4-6h.

Recombinant human activated protein C
-Drotrecogin alfa, (Xigris), 24 mg/kg/h IV infusion for 96 hours.

Blood Pressure Support
-Dopamine 4-20 mcg/kg/min (400 mg in 250 cc D5W, 1600 mcg/mL).
-Norepinephrine 2-8 mcg/min IV infusion (8 mg in 250 mL D5W).
-Albumin 25 gm IV (100 mL of 25% sln) **OR**
-Hetastarch (Hespan) 500-1000 cc over 30-60 min (max 1500 cc/d).
-Dobutamine 5 mcg/kg/min, and titrate to bp keep systolic BP >90 mmHg; max
  10 mcg/kg/min.

10. Symptomatic Medications:
-Acetaminophen (Tylenol) 650 mg PR q4-6h prn temp >39°C.
-Famotidine (Pepcid) 20 mg IV/PO q12h.
-Heparin 5000 U SQ q12h or pneumatic compression stockings.
-Docusate sodium 100-200 mg PO qhs.

11. Extras: CXR, KUB, ECG. Ultrasound, lumbar puncture.

12. Labs: CBC with differential, SMA 7&12, blood C&S x 3, T&C for 3-6 units
  PRBC, INR/PTT, drug levels peak and trough at 3rd dose. UA. Cultures of
  urine, sputum, wound, IV catheters, decubitus ulcers, pleural fluid.

Peritonitis

1. **Admit to:**
2. **Diagnosis:** Peritonitis
3. **Condition:**
4. **Vital Signs:** q1-6h. Call physician if BP >160/90, <90/60; P >120, <50; R>25, <10; T >38.5°C.
5. **Activity:** Bed rest.
6. **Nursing:** Guaiac stools.
7. **Diet:** NPO
8. **IV Fluids:** D5 ½ NS at 125 cc/h.
9. **Special Medications:**

Primary Bacterial Peritonitis -- Spontaneous:

Option 1:
   -Ampicillin 1-2 gm IV q 4-6h (vancomycin 1 gm IV q12h if penicillin allergic)
      AND EITHER
   Cefotaxime (Claforan) 1-2 gm IV q6h **OR**
   Ceftizoxime (Cefizox) 1-2 gm IV q8h **OR**
   Gentamicin or tobramycin 1.5 mg/kg IV, then 1 mg/kg q8h or 7 mg/kg in 50 mL of D5W over 60 min IV q24h.

Option 2:
   -Ticarcillin/clavulanate (Timentin) 3.1 gm IV q6h **OR**
   -Piperacillin/tazobactam (Zosyn) 3.375 gm IV q6h **OR**
   -Imipenem/cilastatin (Primaxin) 0.5-1.0 gm IV q6h **OR**
   -Meropenem (Merrem) 500-1000 mg IV q8h.

Secondary Bacterial Peritonitis – Abdominal Perforation or Rupture:

Option 1:
   -Ampicillin 1-2 gm IV q4-6h **AND**
   Gentamicin or tobramycin as above **AND**
   Metronidazole (Flagyl) 500 mg IV q8h **OR**
   Cefoxitin (Mefoxin) 1-2 gm IV q6h **OR**
   Cefotetan (Cefotan) 1-2 gm IV q12h.

Option 2:
   -Ticarcillin/clavulanate (Timentin) 3.1 gm IV q4-6h (200-300 mg/kg/d) with an aminoglycoside as above **OR**
   -Piperacillin/tazobactam (Zosyn) 3.375 gm IV q6h with an aminoglycoside as above **OR**
   -Ampicillin/sulbactam (Unasyn) 1.5-3.0 gm IV q6h with aminoglycoside as above **OR**
   -Imipenem/cilastatin (Primaxin) 0.5-1.0 gm IV q6-8h **OR**
   -Meropenem (Merrem) 500-1000 mg IV q8h.

Fungal Peritonitis:
   -Amphotericin B peritoneal dialysis, 2 mg/L of dialysis fluid over the first 24 hours, then 1.5 mg in each liter **OR**
   -Fluconazole (Diflucan) 200 mg IV x 1, then 100 mg IV qd.

10. **Symptomatic Medications:**
   -Famotidine (Pepcid) 20 mg IV/PO q12h.
   -Acetaminophen (Tylenol) 325 mg PO/PR q4-6h prn temp >38.5°C.
   -Heparin 5000 U SQ q12h.
11. **Extras:** Plain film, upright abdomen, lateral decubitus, CXR PA and LAT; surgery consult; ECG, abdominal ultrasound. CT scan.
12. **Labs:** CBC with differential, SMA 7&12, amylase, lactate, INR/PTT, UA with

micro, C&S; drug levels peak and trough 3rd dose.

Paracentesis Tube 1: Cell count and differential (1-2 mL, EDTA purple top tube)

Tube 2: Gram stain of sediment; inject 10-20 mL into anaerobic and aerobic culture bottle; AFB, fungal C&S (3-4 mL).

Tube 3: Glucose, protein, albumin, LDH, triglycerides, specific gravity, bilirubin, amylase (2-3 mL, red top tube).

Syringe: pH, lactate (3 mL).

Diverticulitis

1. **Admit to:**
2. **Diagnosis:** Diverticulitis
3. **Condition:**
4. **Vital Signs:** qid. Call physician if BP systolic >160/90, <90/60; P >120, <50; R>25, <10; T >38.5°C
5. **Activity:** Up ad lib.
6. **Nursing:** Inputs and outputs.
7. **Diet:** NPO. Advance to clear liquids as tolerated.
8. **IV Fluids:** 0.5-2 L NS over 1-2 hr then, D5 ½ NS at 125 cc/hr. NG tube at low intermittent suction (if obstructed).
9. **Special Medications:**

Regimen 1:
   -Gentamicin or tobramycin 100-120 mg IV (1.5-2 mg/kg), then 80 mg IV q8h (5 mg/kg/d) or 7 mg/kg in 50 mL of D5W over 60 min IV q24h **AND EITHER**

   Cefoxitin (Mefoxin) 2 gm IV q6-8h **OR**

   Clindamycin (Cleocin) 600-900 mg IV q8h.

Regimen 2:
   -Metronidazole (Flagyl) 500 mg q8h **AND**

   Ciprofloxacin (Cipro) 250-500 mg PO bid or 200-300 mg IV q12h.

Outpatient Regimen:
   -Metronidazole (Flagyl) 500 mg PO q6h **AND EITHER**

   Ciprofloxacin (Cipro) 500 mg PO bid **OR**

   Trimethoprim/SMX (Bactrim) 1 DS tab PO bid.

10. **Symptomatic Medications:**
   -Meperidine (Demerol) 50-100 mg IM or IV q3-4h prn pain.

   -Zolpidem (Ambien) 5-10 mg qhs prn insomnia.

11. **Extras:** Acute abdomen series, CXR PA and LAT, ECG, CT scan of abdomen, ultrasound, surgery and GI consults.
12. **Labs:** CBC with differential, SMA 7&12, amylase, lipase, blood cultures x 2, drug levels peak and trough 3rd dose. UA, C&S.

Lower Urinary Tract Infection

1. **Admit to:**
2. **Diagnosis:** UTI.
3. **Condition:**
4. **Vital Signs:** q shift. Call physician if BP <90/60; >160/90; R >30, <10; P >120, <50; T >38.5°C
5. **Activity:** Up ad lib
6. **Nursing:**
7. **Diet:** Regular
8. **IV Fluids:**
9. **Special Medications:**

Lower Urinary Tract Infection (treat for 3-7 days):
   - Trimethoprim-sulfamethoxazole (Septra) 1 double strength tab (160/800 mg) PO bid.
   - Norfloxacin (Noroxin) 400 mg PO bid.
   - Ciprofloxacin (Cipro) 250 mg PO bid.
   - Levofloxacin (Levaquin) 500 mg IV/PO q24h.
   - Lomefloxacin (Maxaquin) 400 mg PO qd.
   - Enoxacin (Penetrex) 200-400 mg PO q12h; 1h before or 2h after meals.
   - Cefpodoxime (Vantin) 100 mg PO bid.
   - Cephalexin (Keflex) 500 mg PO q6h.
   - Cefixime (Suprax) 200 mg PO q12h or 400 mg PO qd.
   - Cefazolin (Ancef) 1-2 gm IV q8h.

Complicated or Catheter-Associated Urinary Tract Infection:
   - Ceftizoxime (Cefizox) 1 gm IV q8h.
   - Gentamicin 2 mg/kg, then 1.5/kg q8h or 7 mg/kg in 50 mL of D5W over 60 min IV q24h.
   - Ticarcillin/clavulanate (Timentin) 3.1 gm IV q4-6h
   - Ciprofloxacin (Cipro) 500 mg PO bid.
   - Levofloxacin (Levaquin) 500 mg IV/PO q24h.

Prophylaxis (≥3 episodes/yr):
   - Trimethoprim/SMX single strength tab PO qhs.

Candida Cystitis
   - Fluconazole (Diflucan) 100 mg PO or IV x 1 dose, then 50 mg PO or IV qd for 5 days **OR**
   - Amphotericin B continuous bladder irrigation, 50 mg/1000 mL sterile water via 3-way Foley catheter at 1 L/d for 5 days.

10. **Symptomatic Medications:**
   - Phenazopyridine (Pyridium) 100 mg PO tid.
   - Docusate sodium (Colace) 100 mg PO qhs.
   - Acetaminophen (Tylenol) 325-650 mg PO q4-6h prn temp >39° C.
   - Zolpidem (Ambien) 5-10 mg qhs prn insomnia.
11. **Extras:** Renal ultrasound.
12. **Labs:** CBC, SMA 7. UA with micro, urine Gram stain, C&S.

Pyelonephritis

1. **Admit to:**
2. **Diagnosis:** Pyelonephritis
3. **Condition:**
4. **Vital Signs:** tid. Call physician if BP <90/60; >160/90; R >30, <10; P >120, <50; T >38.5°C
5. **Activity:**
6. **Nursing:** Inputs and outputs.
7. **Diet:** Regular
8. **IV Fluids:** D5 ½ NS at 125 cc/h.
9. **Special Medications:**
   - Trimethoprim-sulfamethoxazole (Septra) 160/800 mg (10 mL in 100 mL D5W IV over 2 hours) q12h or 1 double strength tab PO bid.
   - Ciprofloxacin (Cipro) 500 mg PO bid or 400 mg IV q12h.
   - Norfloxacin (Noroxin) 400 mg PO bid
   - Ofloxacin (Floxin) 400 mg PO or IV bid.
   - Levofloxacin (Levaquin) 500 mg PO/IV q24h.
   - In more severely ill patients, treatment with an IV third-generation cephalosporin, or ticarcillin/clavulanic acid, or piperacillin/tazobactam or imipenem is recommended with an aminoglycoside.
   - Ceftizoxime (Cefizox) 1 gm IV q8h.
   - Ceftazidime (Fortaz) 1 gm IV q8h.
   - Ticarcillin/clavulanate (Timentin) 3.1 gm IV q6h.
   - Piperacillin/tazobactam (Zosyn) 3.375 gm IV/PB q6h.
   - Imipenem/cilastatin (Primaxin) 0.5-1.0 gm IV q6-8h.
   - Gentamicin or tobramycin, 2 mg/kg IV, then 1.5 mg/kg q8h or 7 mg/kg in 50 mL of D5W over 60 min IV q24h.
10. **Symptomatic Medications:**
    - Phenazopyridine (Pyridium) 100 mg PO tid.
    - Meperidine (Demerol) 50-100 mg IM q4-6h prn pain.
    - Docusate sodium (Colace) 100 mg PO qhs.
    - Acetaminophen (Tylenol) 325-650 mg PO q4-6h prn temp >39° C.
    - Zolpidem (Ambien) 5-10 mg qhs prn insomnia.
11. **Extras:** Renal ultrasound, KUB.
12. **Labs:** CBC with differential, SMA 7. UA with micro, urine Gram stain, C&S; blood C&S x 2. Drug levels peak and trough third dose third dose.

Osteomyelitis

1. **Admit to:**
2. **Diagnosis:** Osteomyelitis
3. **Condition:**
4. **Vital Signs:** qid. Call physician if BP <90/60; T >38.5°C
5. **Activity:** Bed rest with bathroom privileges.
6. **Nursing:** Keep involved extremity elevated. Range of motion exercises tid.
7. **Diet:** Regular, high fiber.
8. **IV Fluids:** Heparin lock with flush q shift.

9. Special Medications:
Adult Empiric Therapy:
-Nafcillin or oxacillin 2 gm IV q4h **OR**
-Cefazolin (Ancef) 1-2 gm IV q8h **OR**
-Vancomycin 1 gm IV q12h (1 gm in 250 cc D5W over 1h).
-**Add** 3rd generation cephalosporin if gram negative bacilli on Gram stain. Treat for 4-6 weeks.

Post-Operative or Post-Trauma:
-Vancomycin 1 gm IV q12h **AND** ceftazidime (Fortaz) 1-2 gm IV q8h.
-Imipenem/cilastatin (Primaxin)**(single-drug treatment)** 0.5-1.0 gm IV q6-8h.
-Ticarcillin/clavulanate (Timentin)**(single-drug treatment)** 3.1 gm IV q4-6h.
-Ciprofloxacin (Cipro) 500-750 mg PO bid or 400 mg IV q12h **AND** Rifampin 600 mg PO qd.

Osteomyelitis with Decubitus Ulcer:
-Cefoxitin (Mefoxin), 2 gm IV q6-8h.
-Ciprofloxacin (Cipro) and metronidazole 500 mg IV q8h.
-Imipenem/cilastatin (Primaxin), see dosage above.
-Nafcillin, gentamicin and clindamycin; see dosage above.

10. Symptomatic Medications:
-Meperidine (Demerol) 50-100 mg IM q3-4h prn pain.
-Docusate sodium (Colace) 100 mg PO qhs.
-Heparin 5000 U SQ bid.

11. Extras: Technetium/gallium bone scans, multiple X-ray views, CT/MRI.
12. Labs: CBC with differential, SMA 7, blood C&S x 3, MIC, MBC, UA with micro, C&S. Needle biopsy of bone for C&S. Trough antibiotic levels.

Active Pulmonary Tuberculosis

1. Admit to:
2. Diagnosis: Active Pulmonary Tuberculosis
3. Condition:
4. Vital Signs: q shift
5. Activity: Up ad lib in room.
6. Nursing: Respiratory isolation.
7. Diet: Regular
8. Special Medications:
-Isoniazid 300 mg PO qd (5 mg/kg/d, max 300 mg/d) **AND** Rifampin 600 mg PO qd (10 mg/kg/d, 600 mg/d max) **AND** Pyrazinamide 500 mg PO bid-tid (15-30 mg/kg/d, max 2.5 gm) **AND** Ethambutol 400 mg PO bid-tid (15-25 mg/kg/d, 2.5 gm/d max).
-Empiric treatment consists of a 4-drug combination of isoniazid (INH), rifampin, pyrazinamide (PZA), and either ethambutol or streptomycin. A modified regimen is recommended for patients known to have INH-resistant TB. Treat for 8 weeks with the four-drug regimen, followed by 18 weeks of INH and rifampin.
-Pyridoxine 50 mg PO qd with INH.

Prophylaxis
-Isoniazid 300 mg PO qd (5 mg/kg/d) x 6-9 months.
9. Extras: CXR PA, LAT, ECG.
10. Labs: CBC with differential, SMA7 and 12, LFTs, HIV serology. First AM sputum for AFB x 3 samples.

Cellulitis

1. Admit to:
2. Diagnosis: Cellulitis
3. Condition:
4. Vital Signs: tid. Call physician if BP <90/60; T >38.5°C
5. Activity: Up ad lib.
6. Nursing: Keep affected extremity elevated; warm compresses prn.
7. Diet: Regular, encourage fluids.
8. IV Fluids: Heparin lock with flush q shift.
9. Special Medications:
Empiric Therapy Cellulitis
   -Nafcillin or oxacillin 1-2 gm IV q4-6h **OR**
   -Cefazolin (Ancef) 1-2 gm IV q8h **OR**
   -Vancomycin 1 gm q12h (1 gm in 250 cc D5W over 1h) **OR**
   -Erythromycin 500 IV/PO q6h **OR**
   -Dicloxacillin 500 mg PO qid; may add penicillin VK, 500 mg PO qid, to
     increase coverage for streptococcus **OR**
   -Cephalexin (Keflex) 500 mg PO qid.
Immunosuppressed, Diabetic Patients, or Ulcerated Lesions:
   -Nafcillin or cefazolin and gentamicin or aztreonam. Add clindamycin or
     metronidazole if septic.
   -Cefoxitin (Ancef) 1-2 gm IV q8h.
   -Cefoxitin (Mefoxin) 1-2 gm IV q6-8h.
   -Gentamicin 2 mg/kg, then 1.5 mg/kg IV q8h or 7 mg/kg in 50 mL of D5W over
     60 min IV q24h **OR** aztreonam (Azactam) 1-2 gm IV q6h **PLUS**
   -Metronidazole (Flagyl) 500 mg IV q8h or clindamycin 900 mg IV q8h.
   -Ticarcillin/clavulanate (Timentin) **(single-drug treatment)** 3.1 gm IV q4-6h.
   -Ampicillin/Sulbactam (Unasyn) **(single-drug therapy)** 1.5-3.0 gm IV q6h.
   -Imipenem/cilastatin (Primaxin) **(single-drug therapy)** 0.5-1 mg IV q6-8h.
10. Symptomatic Medications:
   -Acetaminophen/codeine (Tylenol #3) 1-2 PO q4-6h prn pain.
   -Docusate sodium (Colace) 100 mg PO qhs.
   -Acetaminophen (Tylenol) 325-650 mg PO q4-6h prn temp >39° C.
   -Zolpidem (Ambien) 5-10 mg qhs prn insomnia.
11. Extras: Technetium/Gallium scans, Doppler study (ankle-brachial indices).
12. Labs: CBC, SMA 7, blood C&S x 2. Leading edge aspirate for Gram stain,
   C&S; UA, antibiotic levels.

Pelvic Inflammatory Disease

1. Admit to:
2. Diagnosis: Pelvic Inflammatory Disease
3. Condition:
4. Vital Signs: q8h. Call physician if BP >160/90, <90/60; P >120, <50; R>25,
   <10; T >38.5°C
5. Activity:
6. Nursing: Inputs and outputs.
7. Diet: Regular

8. IV Fluids: D5 ½ NS at 100-125 cc/hr.

9. Special Medications:
-Cefoxitin (Mefoxin) 2 gm IV q6h **OR** cefotetan (Cefotan) 1-2 gm IV q12h;
   AND doxycycline (Vibramycin) 100 mg IV q12h (IV for 4 days and 48h after
   afebrile, then complete 10-14 days of doxycycline 100 mg PO bid) **OR**
-Clindamycin 900 mg IV q8h **AND** Gentamicin 2 mg/kg IV, then 1.5 mg/kg IV
   q8h or 7 mg/kg in 50 mL of D5W over 60 min IV q24h, then complete 10-
   14 d of Clindamycin 300 mg PO qid or Doxycycline 100 mg PO bid **OR**
-Ceftriaxone (Rocephin) 250 mg IM x 1 and doxycycline 100 mg PO bid for 14
   days **OR**
-Ofloxacin (Floxin) 400 mg PO bid for 14 days.

AND EITHER
-Clindamycin 300 mg PO qid for 14 days **OR**
-Metronidazole (Flagyl) 500 mg PO bid for 14 days.

10. Symptomatic Medications:
-Acetaminophen (Tylenol) 1-2 tabs PO q4-6h prn pain or temperature
   >38.5°C.
-Meperidine (Demerol) 25-100 mg IM q4-6h prn pain.
-Zolpidem (Ambien) 10 mg PO qhs prn insomnia.

11. Labs: CBC, SMA 7&12, ESR. GC culture, chlamydia direct fluorescent
antibody stain. UA with micro, C&S, VDRL, HIV, blood cultures x 2. Pelvic
ultrasound.

Gastrointestinal Disorders

Gastroesophageal Reflux Disease

1. **Admit to:**
2. **Diagnosis:** Gastroesophageal reflux disease.
3. **Condition:**
4. **Vital Signs:** q4h. Call physician if BP >160/90, <90/60; P >120, <50; T >38.5°C
5. **Activity:** Up ad lib. Elevate the head of the bed by 6 to 8 inches.
6. **Nursing:** Guaiac stools.
7. **Diet:** Low-fat diet; no cola, citrus juices, or tomato products; avoid the supine position after meals; no eating within 3 hours of bedtime.
8. **IV Fluids:** D5 ½ NS with 20 mEq KCL at TKO.
9. **Special Medications:**
   -Pantoprazole (Protonix) 40 mg PO/IV q24h **OR**
   -Nizatidine (Axid) 300 mg PO qhs **OR**
   -Omeprazole (Prilosec) 20 mg PO bid (30 minutes prior to meals) **OR**
   -Lansoprazole (Prevacid) 15-30 mg PO qd prior to breakfast [15, 30 mg caps] **OR**
   -Esomeprazole (Nexium) 20 or 40 mg PO qd **OR**
   -Rabeprazole (Aciphex) 20 mg delayed-release tablet PO qd **OR**
   -Ranitidine (Zantac) 50 mg IV bolus, then continuous infusion at 12.5 mg/h (300 mg in 250 mL D5W at 11 mL/h over 24h) or 50 mg IV q8h **OR**
   -Cimetidine (Tagamet) 300 mg IV bolus, then continuous infusion at 50 mg/h (1200 mg in 250 mL D5W over 24h) or 300 mg IV q6-8h **OR**
   -Famotidine (Pepcid) 20 mg IV q12h.
10. **Symptomatic Medications:**
    -Trimethobenzamide (Tigan) 100-250 mg PO or 100-200 mg IM/PR q6h prn nausea **OR**
    -Prochlorperazine (Compazine) 5-10 mg IM/IV/PO q4-6h or 25 mg PR q4-6h prn nausea.
11. **Extras:** Upright abdomen, KUB, CXR, ECG, endoscopy. GI consult, surgery consult.
12. **Labs:** CBC, SMA 7&12, amylase, lipase, LDH. UA.

Peptic Ulcer Disease

1. **Admit to:**
2. **Diagnosis:** Peptic ulcer disease.
3. **Condition:**
4. **Vital Signs:** q4h. Call physician if BP >160/90, <90/60; P >120, <50; T >38.5°C
5. **Activity:** Up ad lib
6. **Nursing:** Guaiac stools.
7. **Diet:** NPO 48h, then regular, no caffeine.
8. **IV Fluids:** D5 ½ NS with 20 mEq KCL at 125 cc/h. NG tube at low intermittent suction (if obstructed).

9. Special Medications:
  -Ranitidine (Zantac) 50 mg IV bolus, then continuous infusion at 12.5 mg/h (300 mg in 250 mL D5W at 11 mL/h over 24h) or 50 mg IV q8h **OR**
  -Cimetidine (Tagamet) 300 mg IV bolus, then continuous infusion at 50 mg/h (1200 mg in 250 mL D5W over 24h) or 300 mg IV q6-8h **OR**
  -Famotidine (Pepcid) 20 mg IV q12h **OR**
  -Pantoprazole (Protonix) 40 mg PO/IV q24h **OR**
  -Nizatidine (Axid) 300 mg PO qhs **OR**
  -Omeprazole (Prilosec) 20 mg PO bid (30 minutes prior to meals) **OR**
  -Lansoprazole (Prevacid) 15-30 mg PO qd prior to breakfast [15, 30 mg caps].

Eradication of Helicobacter pylori
  A. Bismuth, Metronidazole, Tetracycline, Ranitidine
    1. 14 day therapy.
    2. Bismuth (Pepto Bismol) 2 tablets PO qid.
    3. Metronidazole (Flagyl) 250 mg PO qid (tid if cannot tolerate the qid dosing).
    4. Tetracycline 500 mg PO qid.
    5. Ranitidine (Zantac) 150 mg PO bid.
    6. Efficacy is greater than 90%.
  B. Amoxicillin, Omeprazole, Clarithromycin (AOC)
    1. 10 days of therapy.
    2. Amoxicillin 1 gm PO bid.
    3. Omeprazole (Prilosec) 20 mg PO bid.
    4. Clarithromycin (Biaxin) 500 mg PO bid.
  C. Metronidazole, Omeprazole, Clarithromycin (MOC)
    1. 10 days of therapy
    2. Metronidazole 500 mg PO bid.
    3. Omeprazole (Prilosec) 20 mg PO bid.
    4. Clarithromycin (Biaxin) 500 mg PO bid.
    5. Efficacy is >80%
    6. Expensive, usually well tolerated.
  D. Omeprazole, Clarithromycin (OC)
    1. 14 days of therapy.
    2. Omeprazole (Prilosec) 40 mg PO qd for 14 days, then 20 mg qd for an additional 14 days of therapy.
    3. Clarithromycin (Biaxin) 500 mg PO tid.
  E. Ranitidine-Bismuth-Citrate, Clarithromycin (RBC-C)
    1. 28 days of therapy.
    2. Ranitidine-bismuth-citrate (Tritec) 400 mg PO bid for 28 days.
    3. Clarithromycin (Biaxin) 500 mg PO tid for 14 days.
    4. Efficacy is 70-80%; expensive

10. Symptomatic Medications:
  -Trimethobenzamide (Tigan) 100-250 mg PO or 100-200 mg IM/PR q6h prn nausea **OR**
  -Prochlorperazine (Compazine) 5-10 mg IM/IV/PO q4-6h or 25 mg PR q4-6h prn nausea.
11. Extras: Upright abdomen, KUB, CXR, ECG, endoscopy. GI consult, surgery consult.
12. Labs: CBC, SMA 7&12, amylase, lipase, LDH. UA, Helicobacter pylori serology. Fasting serum gastrin qAM for 3 days. Urea breath test for H pylori.

Gastrointestinal Bleeding

1. **Admit to:**
2. **Diagnosis:** Upper/lower GI bleed
3. **Condition:**
4. **Vital Signs:** q30min. Call physician if BP >160/90, <90/60; P >120, <50; R>25, <10; T >38.5°C; urine output <15 mL/hr for 4h.
5. **Activity:** Bed rest
6. **Nursing:** Place nasogastric tube, then lavage with 2 L of room temperature normal saline, then connect to low intermittent suction. Repeat lavage q1h. Record volume and character of lavage. Foley to closed drainage; inputs and outputs.
7. **Diet:** NPO
8. **IV Fluids:** Two 16 gauge IV lines. 1-2 L NS wide open; transfuse 2-6 units PRBC to run as fast as possible, then repeat CBC.
9. **Special Medications:**
   -Oxygen 2 L by NC.
   -Ranitidine (Zantac) 50 mg IV bolus, then continuous infusion at 12.5 mg/h [300 mg in 250 mL D5W over 24h (11 cc/h)], or 50 mg IV q6-8h **OR**
   -Famotidine (Pepcid) 20 mg IV q12h.
   -Vitamin K (Phytonadione) 10 mg IV/SQ qd for 3 days (if INR is elevated).

Esophageal Variceal Bleeds:
   -Somatostatin (Octreotide) 50 mcg IV bolus, followed by 25-50 mcg/h IV infusion (1200 mcg in 250 mL of D5W at 11 mL/h).

   Vasopressin/Nitroglycerine Paste Therapy:
   -Vasopressin (Pitressin) 20 U IV over 20-30 minutes, then 0.2-0.3 U/min [100 U in 250 mL of D5W (0.4 U/mL)] for 30 min, followed by increases of 0.2 U/min until bleeding stops or max of 0.9 U/min. If bleeding stops, taper over 24-48h **AND**
   -Nitroglycerine paste 1 inch q6h **OR** nitroglycerin IV at 10-30 mcg/min continuous infusion (50 mg in 250 mL of D5W).

10. **Extras:** Portable CXR, upright abdomen, ECG. Surgery and GI consults.

Upper GI Bleeds: Esophagogastroduodenoscopy with coagulation or sclerotherapy; Linton-Nachlas tube for tamponade of esophageal varices.

Lower GI Bleeds: Sigmoidoscopy/colonoscopy (after a GoLytely purge 6-8 L over 4-6h), technetium 99m RBC scan, angiography with embolization.

11. **Labs:** Repeat hematocrit q2h; CBC with platelets q12-24h. Repeat INR in 6 hours. SMA 7&12, ALT, AST, alkaline phosphatase, INR/PTT, type and cross for 3-6 U PRBC and 2-4 U FFP.

Cirrhotic Ascites and Edema

1. **Admit to:**
2. **Diagnosis:** Cirrhotic ascites and edema
3. **Condition:**
4. **Vital Signs:** Vitals q4-6 hours. Call physician if BP >160/90, <90/60; P >120, <50; T >38.5°C; urine output < 25 cc/hr for 4h.
5. **Activity:** Bed rest with legs elevated.
6. **Nursing:** Inputs and outputs, daily weights, measure abdominal girth qd, guaiac all stools.

7. **Diet:** 2500 calories, 100 gm protein; 500 mg sodium restriction; fluid restriction to 1-1.5 L/d (if hyponatremia, Na <130).
8. **IV Fluids:** Heparin lock with flush q shift.
9. **Special Medications:**
   -Diurese to reduce weight by 0.5-1 kg/d (if edema) or 0.25 kg/d (if no edema).
   -Spironolactone (Aldactone) 25-50 mg PO qid or 200 mg PO qAM, increase by 100 mg/d to max of 400 mg/d.
   -Furosemide (Lasix)(refractory ascites) 40-120 mg PO or IV qd-bid. Add KCL 20-40 mEq PO qAM if renal function is normal **OR**
   -Torsemide (Demadex) 20-40 mg PO/IV qd-bid.
   -Metolazone (Zaroxolyn) 5-10 mg PO qd (max 20 mg/d).
   -Famotidine (Pepcid) 20 mg IV/PO q12h.
   -Vitamin K 10 mg SQ qd for 3d.
   -Folic acid 1 mg PO qd.
   -Thiamine 100 mg PO qd.
   -Multivitamin PO qd.

   Paracentesis: Remove up to 5 L of ascites if peripheral edema, tense ascites, or decreased diaphragmatic excursion. If large volume paracentesis without peripheral edema or with renal insufficiency, give salt-poor albumin, 12.5 gm for each 2 liters of fluid removed (50 mL of 25% solution); infuse 25 mL before paracentesis and 25 mL 6h after.

10. **Symptomatic Medications:**
    -Docusate sodium (Colace) 100 mg PO qhs.
    -Lactulose 30 mL PO bid-qid prn constipation.
    -Acetaminophen (Tylenol) 325-650 mg PO q4-6h prn headache.
11. **Extras:** KUB, CXR, abdominal ultrasound, liver-spleen scan, GI consult.
12. **Labs:** Ammonia, CBC, SMA 7&12, LFTs, albumin, amylase, lipase, INR/PTT. Urine creatinine, Na, K. HBsAg, anti-HBs, hepatitis C virus antibody, alpha-1-antitrypsin.

Paracentesis Ascitic Fluid

   Tube 1: Protein, albumin, specific gravity, glucose, bilirubin, amylase, lipase, triglyceride, LDH (3-5 mL, red top tube).

   Tube 2: Cell count and differential (3-5 mL, purple top tube).

   Tube 3: C&S, Gram stain, AFB, fungal (5-20 mL); inject 20 mL into bottle of blood culture at bedside.

   Tube 4: Cytology (>20 mL).

   Syringe: pH (2 mL).

Viral Hepatitis

1. **Admit to:**
2. **Diagnosis:** Hepatitis
3. **Condition:**
4. **Vital Signs:** qid. Call physician if BP <90/60; T >38.5°C
5. **Activity:**
6. **Nursing:** Stool isolation.
7. **Diet:** Clear liquid (if nausea), low fat (if diarrhea).
8. **Special Medications:**
   -Famotidine (Pepcid) 20 mg IV/PO q12h.
   -Vitamin K 10 mg SQ qd for 3d.
   -Multivitamin PO qd.

9. Symptomatic Medications:
-Meperidine (Demerol) 50-100 mg IM q4-6h prn pain.
-Trimethobenzamide (Tigan) 250 mg PO q6-8h prn pruritus or nausea q6-8h prn.
-Hydroxyzine (Vistaril) 25 mg IM/PO q4-6h prn pruritus or nausea.
-Diphenhydramine (Benadryl) 25-50 mg PO/IV q4-6h prn pruritus.
10. Extras: Ultrasound, GI consult.
11. Labs: CBC, SMA 7&12, GGT, LDH, amylase, lipase, INR/PTT, IgM anti-HAV, IgM anti-HBc, HBsAg, anti-HCV; alpha-1-antitrypsin, ANA, ferritin, ceruloplasmin, urine copper.

Cholecystitis and Cholangitis

1. Admit to:
2. Diagnosis: Bacterial cholangitis
3. Condition:
4. Vital Signs: q4h. Call physician if BP systolic >160, <90; diastolic. >90, <60; P >120, <50; R>25, <10; T >38.5°C
5. Activity: Bed rest
6. Nursing: Inputs and outputs
7. Diet: NPO
8. IV Fluids: 0.5-1 L LR over 1h, then D5 ½ NS with 20 mEq KCL/L at 125 cc/h. NG tube at low constant suction. Foley to closed drainage.
9. Special Medications:
-Ticarcillin or piperacillin 3 gm IV q4-6h, and either metronidazole (Flagyl) 500 mg q8h or cefoxitin (Mefoxin) 1-2 gm IV q6h.
-Ampicillin 1-2 gm IV q4-6h and gentamicin 100 mg (1.5-2 mg/kg), then 80 mg IV q8h (3-5 mg/kg/d) and metronidazole 500 mg IV q8h.
-Imipenem/cilastatin (Primaxin) 1.0 gm IV q6h (single agent).
-Ampicillin/sulbactam (Unasyn) 1.5-3.0 gm IV q6h (single-agent).
10. Symptomatic Medications:
-Meperidine (Demerol) 50-100 mg IV/IM q4-6h prn pain.
-Hydroxyzine (Vistaril) 25-50 mg IV/IM q4-6h prn with meperidine.
-Omeprazole (Prilosec) 20 mg PO bid.
-Heparin 5000 U SQ q12h.
11. Extras: CXR, ECG, RUQ ultrasound, HIDA scan, acute abdomen series. GI consult, surgical consult.
12. Labs: CBC, SMA 7&12, GGT, amylase, lipase, blood C&S x 2. UA, INR/PTT.

Acute Pancreatitis

1. **Admit to:**
2. **Diagnosis:** Acute pancreatitis
3. **Condition:**
4. **Vital Signs:** q1-4h, call physician if BP >160/90, <90/60; P >120, <50; R>25, <10; T >38.5°C; urine output < 25 cc/hr for more than 4 hours.
5. **Activity:** Bed rest with bedside commode.
6. **Nursing:** Inputs and outputs, fingerstick glucose qid, guaiac stools. Foley to closed drainage.
7. **Diet:** NPO
8. **IV Fluids:** 1-4 L NS over 1-3h, then D5 ½ NS with 20 mEq KCL/L at 125 cc/hr. NG tube at low constant suction (if obstruction).
9. **Special Medications:**
   -Ranitidine (Zantac) 6.25 mg/h (150 mg in 250 mL D5W at 11 mL/h) IV or 50 mg IV q6-8h **OR**
   Famotidine (Pepcid) 20 mg IV q12h.
   -Ticarcillin/clavulanate (Timentin) 3.1 gm IV, or ampicillin/sulbactam (Unasyn) 3.0 gm IV q6h or imipenem (Primaxin) 0.5-1.0 gm IV q6h.
   -Antibiotics are indicated for infected pancreatic pseudocysts or for abscess. Uncomplicated pancreatitis does not require antibiotics.
   -Heparin 5000 U SQ q12h.
   -Total parenteral nutrition should be provided until the amylase and lipase are normal and symptoms have resolved.
10. **Symptomatic Medications:**
    -Meperidine 50-100 mg IM/IV q3-4h prn pain.
11. **Extras:** Upright abdomen, portable CXR, ECG, ultrasound, CT with contrast. Surgery and GI consults.
12. **Labs:** CBC, platelets, SMA 7&12, calcium, triglycerides, amylase, lipase, LDH, AST, ALT; blood C&S x 2, hepatitis B surface antigen, INR/PTT, type and hold 4-6 U PRBC and 2-4 U FFP. UA.

Acute Diarrhea

1. **Admit to:**
2. **Diagnosis:** Acute Diarrhea
3. **Condition:**
4. **Vital Signs:** q6h; call physician if BP >160/90, <80/60; P >120; R>25; T >38.5°C
5. **Activity:** Up ad lib
6. **Nursing:** Daily weights, inputs and outputs.
7. **Diet:** NPO except ice chips for 24h, then low residual elemental diet; no milk products.
8. **IV Fluids:** 1-2 L NS over 1-2 hours; then D5 ½ NS with 40 mEq KCL/L at 125 cc/h.
9. **Special Medications:**
Febrile or gross blood in stool or neutrophils on microscopic exam or prior travel:
   -Ciprofloxacin (Cipro) 500 mg PO bid **OR**
   -Levofloxacin (Levaquin) 500 mg PO qd **OR**

-Trimethoprim/SMX (Bactrim DS) (160/800 mg) one DS tab PO bid.

11. Extras: Upright abdomen. GI consult.

12. Labs: SMA7 and 12, CBC with differential, UA, blood culture x 2.

Stool studies: Wright's stain for fecal leukocytes, ova and parasites x 3, clostridium difficile toxin, culture for enteric pathogens, E coli 0157:H7 culture.

Specific Treatment of Acute Diarrhea

Shigella:
-Trimethoprim/SMX, (Bactrim) one DS tab PO bid for 5 days **OR**
-Ciprofloxacin (Cipro) 500 mg PO bid for 5 days **OR**
-Azithromycin (Zithromax) 500 mg PO x 1, then 250 mg PO qd x 4.

Salmonella (bacteremia):
-Ofloxacin (Floxin) 400 mg IV/PO q12h for 14 days **OR**
-Ciprofloxacin (Cipro) 400 mg IV q12h or 750 mg PO q12h for 14 days **OR**
-Trimethoprim/SMX (Bactrim) one DS tab PO bid for 14 days **OR**
-Ceftriaxone (Rocephin) 2 gm IV q12h for 14 days.

Campylobacter jejuni:
-Erythromycin 250 mg PO qid for 5-10 days **OR**
-Azithromycin (Zithromax) 500 mg PO x 1, then 250 mg PO qd x 4 **OR**
-Ciprofloxacin (Cipro) 500 mg PO bid for 5 days.

Enterotoxic/Enteroinvasive E coli (Travelers Diarrhea):
-Ciprofloxacin (Cipro) 500 mg PO bid for 5-7 days **OR**
-Trimethoprim/SMX (Bactrim), one DS tab PO bid for 5-7 days.

Antibiotic-Associated and Pseudomembranous Colitis (Clostridium difficile):
-Metronidazole (Flagyl) 250 mg PO or IV qid for 10-14 days **OR**
-Vancomycin 125 mg PO qid for 10 days (500 PO qid for 10-14 days, if recurrent).

Yersinia Enterocolitica (sepsis):
-Trimethoprim/SMX (Bactrim), one DS tab PO bid for 5-7 days **OR**
-Ciprofloxacin (Cipro) 500 mg PO bid for 5-7 days **OR**
-Ofloxacin (Floxin) 400 mg PO bid **OR**
-Ceftriaxone (Rocephin) 1 gm IV q12h.

Entamoeba Histolytica (Amebiasis):
Mild to Moderate Intestinal Disease:
-Metronidazole (Flagyl) 750 mg PO tid for 10 days **OR**
-Tinidazole 2 gm per day PO for 3 days **Followed By:**
-Iodoquinol 650 mg PO tid for 20 days **OR**
-Paromomycin 25-30 mg/kg/d PO tid for 7 days.

Severe Intestinal Disease:
-Metronidazole (Flagyl)750 mg PO tid for 10 days **OR**
-Tinidazole 600 mg PO bid for 5 days **Followed By:**
-Iodoquinol 650 mg PO tid for 20 days **OR**
-Paromomycin 25-30 mg/kg/d PO tid for 7 days.

Giardia Lamblia:
-Quinacrine 100 mg PO tid for 5d **OR**
-Metronidazole 250 mg PO tid for 7 days.

Cryptosporidium:
-Paromomycin 500 mg PO qid for 7-10 days [250 mg].

Crohn's Disease

1. **Admit to:**
2. **Diagnosis:** Crohn's disease.
3. **Condition:**
4. **Vital Signs:** q8h. Call physician if BP >160/90, <90/60; P >120, <50; R>25, <10; T >38.5°C
5. **Activity:** Up ad lib in room.
6. **Nursing:** Inputs and outputs. NG at low intermittent suction (if obstruction).
7. **Diet:** NPO except for ice chips and medications for 48h, then low residue or elemental diet, no milk products.
8. **IV Fluids:** 1-2 L NS over 1-3h, then D5 ½ NS with 40 mEq KCL/L at 125 cc/hr.
9. **Special Medications:**
   -Mesalamine (Asacol) 400-800 mg PO tid or mesalamine (Pentasa) 1000 mg (four 250 mg tabs) PO qid **OR**
   -Sulfasalazine (Azulfidine) 0.5-1 gm PO bid; increase over 10 days to 0.5-1 gm PO qid **OR**
   -Olsalazine (Dipentum) 500 mg PO bid.
   -Infliximab (Remicade) 5 mg/kg IV over 2 hours; MR at 2 and 6 weeks
   -Prednisone 40-60 mg/d PO in divided doses **OR**
   -Hydrocortisone 50-100 mg IV q6h **OR**
   -Methylprednisolone (Solu-Medrol) 10-20 mg IV q6h.
   -Metronidazole (Flagyl) 250-500 mg PO q6h.
   -Vitamin B_{12}, 100 mcg IM for 5d then 100-200 mcg IM q month.
   -Multivitamin PO qAM or 1 ampule IV qAM.
   -Folic acid 1 mg PO qd.
10. **Extras:** Abdominal x-ray series, CXR, colonoscopy. GI consult.
11. **Labs:** CBC, SMA 7&12, Mg, ionized calcium, blood C&S x 2; stool Wright's stain, stool culture, C difficile antigen assay, stool ova and parasites x 3.

Ulcerative Colitis

1. **Admit to:**
2. **Diagnosis:** Ulcerative colitis
3. **Condition:**
4. **Vital Signs:** q4-6h. Call physician if BP >160/90, <90/60; P >120, <50; R>25, <10; T >38.5°C
5. **Activity:** Up ad lib in room.
6. **Nursing:** Inputs and outputs.
7. **Diet:** NPO except for ice chips for 48h, then low residue or elemental diet, no milk products.
8. **IV Fluids:** 1-2 L NS over 1-2h, then D5 ½ NS with 40 mEq KCL/L at 125 cc/hr.
9. **Special Medications:**
   -Mesalamine (Asacol) 400-800 mg PO tid **OR**
   -5-aminosalicylate (Mesalamine) 400-800 mg PO tid or 1 gm PO qid or enema 4 gm/60 mL PR qhs **OR**
   -Sulfasalazine (Azulfidine) 0.5-1 gm PO bid, increase over 10 days as tolerated to 0.5-1.0 gm PO qid **OR**
   -Olsalazine (Dipentum) 500 mg PO bid **OR**
   -Hydrocortisone retention enema, 100 mg in 120 mL saline bid.

-Methylprednisolone (Solu-Medrol) 10-20 mg IV q6h **OR**
-Hydrocortisone 100 mg IV q6h **OR**
-Prednisone 40-60 mg/d PO in divided doses.
-B12, 100 mcg IM for 5d then 100-200 mcg IM q month.
-Multivitamin PO qAM or 1 ampule IV qAM.
-Folate 1 mg PO qd.

10. Symptomatic Medications:
-Loperamide (Imodium) 2-4 mg PO tid-qid prn, max 16 mg/d **OR**
-Kaopectate 60-90 mL PO qid prn.

11. Extras: Upright abdomen. CXR, colonoscopy, GI consult.

12. Labs: CBC, SMA 7&12, Mg, ionized calcium, liver panel, blood C&S x 2; stool Wright's stain, stool for ova and parasites x 3, culture for enteric pathogens; Clostridium difficile antigen assay, UA.

Parenteral Nutrition

General Considerations: Daily weights, inputs and outputs. Finger stick glucose q6h.

Central Parenteral Nutrition:
-Infuse 40-50 mL/h of amino acid-dextrose solution in the first 24h; increase daily by 40 mL/hr increments until providing 1.3-2 x basal energy requirement and 1.2-1.7 gm protein/kg/d (see formula page 97).

Standard solution:

Amino acid sln (Aminosyn) 7-10%	500 mL
Dextrose 40-70%	500 mL
Sodium	35 mEq
Potassium	36 mEq
Chloride	35 mEq
Calcium	4.5 mEq
Phosphate	9 mmol
Magnesium	8.0 mEq
Acetate	82-104 mEq
Multi-trace element formula (zinc, copper, manganese, chromium)	1 mL/d
Regular insulin (if indicated)	10-60 U/L
Multivitamin(12)(2 amp)	10 mL/d
Vitamin K (in solution, SQ, IM)	10 mg/week
Vitamin B12	1000 mcg/week
Selenium (after 20 days of continuous TPN)	80 mcg/d

Intralipid 20%, 500 mL/d IVPB; infuse in parallel with standard solution at 1 mL/min for 15 min; if no adverse reactions, increase to 100 mL/hr once daily or 20 mg/hr continuously. Obtain serum triglyceride 6h after end of infusion (maintain <250 mg/dL).

Cyclic Total Parenteral Nutrition:
-12h night schedule; taper continuous infusion in morning by reducing rate to half of original rate for 1 hour. Further reduce rate by half for an additional hour, then discontinue. Finger stick glucose q4-6h; restart TPN in afternoon. Taper at beginning and end of cycle. Final rate of 185 mL/hr for 9-10 h and 2 hours of taper at each end for total of 2000 mL.

Peripheral Parenteral Supplementation:
  -3% amino acid sln (ProCalamine) up to 3 L/d at 125 cc/h **OR**
  -Combine 500 mL amino acid solution 7% or 10% (Aminosyn) and 500 mL
      20% dextrose and electrolyte additive. Infuse at up to 100 cc/hr in
      parallel with:
  -Intralipid 10% or 20% at 1 mL/min for 15 min (test dose); if no adverse
      reactions, infuse 500 mL/d at 21 mL/h over 24h, or up to 100 mL/h over
      5 hours daily.
  -Draw triglyceride level 6h after end of Intralipid infusion.
7. Special Medications:
  -Famotidine 20 mg IV q12h or 40 mg/day in TPN **OR**
  -Ranitidine (Zantac) 50 mg IV q8h or 150 mg/day in TPN.
8. Extras: Nutrition consult.
9. Labs:
  Daily labs: SMA7, osmolality, CBC, cholesterol, triglyceride, urine glucose
      and specific gravity.
  Twice weekly Labs: Calcium, phosphate, SMA-12, magnesium
  Weekly Labs: Serum albumin and protein, pre-albumin, ferritin, INR/PTT,
      zinc, copper, B12, folate, 24h urine nitrogen and creatinine.

Enteral Nutrition

General Considerations: Daily weights, inputs and outputs, nasoduodenal
feeding tube. Head-of-bed at 30° while enteral feeding and 2 hours after
completion.
Enteral Bolus Feeding: Give 50-100 mL of enteral solution (Pulmocare, Jevity,
Vivonex, Osmolite, Vital HN) q3h. Increase amount in 50 mL steps to max of
250-300 mL q3-4h; 30 kcal of nonprotein calories/kg/d and 1.5 gm
protein/kg/d. Before each feeding measure residual volume, and delay
feeding by 1h if >100 mL. Flush tube with 100 cc of water after each bolus.
Continuous enteral infusion: Initial enteral solution (Pulmocare, Jevity,
Vivonex, Osmolite) 30 mL/hr. Measure residual volume q1h for 12h then tid;
hold feeding for 1h if >100 mL. Increase rate by 25-50 mL/hr at 24 hr intervals
as tolerated until final rate of 50-100 mL/hr. Three tablespoonfuls of protein
powder (Promix) may be added to each 500 cc of solution. Flush tube with
100 cc water q8h.
Special Medications:
  -Metoclopramide (Reglan) 10-20 mg IV/NG **OR**
  -Erythromycin 125 mg IV or via nasogastric tube q8h.
  -Famotidine (Pepcid) 20 mg IV/PO q12h **OR**
  -Ranitidine (Zantac 150 mg NG bid.
Symptomatic Medications:
  -Loperamide (Imodium) 2-4 mg NG/J-tube q6h prn, max 16 mg/d **OR**
  -Diphenoxylate/atropine (Lomotil) 1-2 tabs or 5-10 mL (2.5 mg/5 mL) PO/J-
      tube q4-6h prn, max 12 tabs/d **OR**
  -Kaopectate 30 cc NG or in J-tube q8h.
Extras: CXR, plain abdominal x-ray for tube placement, nutrition consult.
Labs:
  Daily labs: SMA7, osmolality, CBC, cholesterol, triglyceride. SMA-12
  Weekly labs when indicated: Protein, Mg, INR/PTT, 24h urine nitrogen and
      creatinine. Pre-albumin, retinol-binding protein.

Hepatic Encephalopathy

1. **Admit to:**
2. **Diagnosis:** Hepatic encephalopathy
3. **Condition:**
4. **Vital Signs:** q1-4h, neurochecks q4h. Call physician if BP >160/90,<90/60; P >120,<50; R>25,<10; T >38.5°C.
5. **Allergies:** Avoid sedatives, NSAIDS or hepatotoxic drugs.
6. **Activity:** Bed rest.
7. **Nursing:** Keep head-of-bed at 40 degrees, guaiac stools; turn patient q2h while awake, chart stools. Seizure precautions, egg crate mattress, soft restraints prn. Record inputs and outputs.
8. **Diet:** NPO for 8 hours, then low-protein nasogastric enteral feedings (Hepatic-Aid II) at 30 mL/hr. Increase rate by 25-50 mL/hr at 24 hr intervals as tolerated until final rate of 50-100 mL/hr as tolerated.
9. **IV Fluids:** D5W at TKO, Foley to closed drainage.
10. **Special Medications:**
    -Sorbitol 70% solution, 30-60 gm PO now.
    -Lactulose 30-45 mL PO q1h for 3 doses, then 15-45 mL PO bid-qid, titrate to produce 3 soft stools/d **OR**
    -Lactulose enema 300 mL added to 700 mL of tap water; instill 200-250 mL per rectal tube bid-qid **AND**
    -Neomycin 1 gm PO q6h (4-12 g/d) **OR**
    -Metronidazole (Flagyl) 250 mg PO q6h.
    -Ranitidine (Zantac) 50 mg IV q8h or 150 mg PO bid **OR**
    -Famotidine (Pepcid) 20 mg IV/PO q12h.
    -Flumazenil (Romazicon) 0.2 mg (2 mL) IV over 30 seconds q1min until a total dose of 3 mg; if a partial response occurs, continue 0.5 mg doses until a total of 5 mg. Flumazenil may help reverse hepatic encephalopathy, even in the absence of benzodiazepine use.
    -Multivitamin PO qAM or 1 ampule IV qAM.
    -Folic acid 1 mg PO/IV qd.
    -Thiamine 100 mg PO/IV qd.
    -Vitamin K 10 mg SQ qd for 3 days if elevated INR.
11. **Extras:** CXR, ECG; GI and dietetics consults.
12. **Labs:** Ammonia, CBC, platelets, SMA 7&12, AST, ALT, GGT, LDH, alkaline phosphatase, protein, albumin, bilirubin, INR/PTT, ABG, blood C&S x 2, hepatitis B surface antibody. UA.

Alcohol Withdrawal

1. **Admit to:**
2. **Diagnosis:** Alcohol withdrawals/delirium tremens.
3. **Condition:**
4. **Vital Signs:** q4-6h. Call physician if BP >160/90, <90/60; P >130, <50; R>25, <10; T >38.5°C; or increase in agitation.
5. **Activity:**
6. **Nursing:** Seizure precautions. Soft restraints prn.
7. **Diet:** Regular, push fluids.
8. **IV Fluids:** Heparin lock or D5 ½ NS at 100-125 cc/h.
9. **Special Medications:**

Withdrawal syndrome:
   -Chlordiazepoxide (Librium) 50-100 mg PO/IV q6h for 3 days **OR**
   -Lorazepam (Ativan) 1 mg PO tid-qid.

Delirium tremens:
   -Chlordiazepoxide (Librium) 100 mg slow IV push or PO, repeat q4-6h prn agitation or tremor for 24h; max 500 mg/d. Then give 50-100 mg PO q6h prn agitation or tremor **OR**
   -Diazepam (Valium) 5 mg slow IV push, repeat q6h until calm, then 5-10 mg PO q4-6h.

Seizures:
   -Thiamine 100 mg IV push **AND**
   -Dextrose water 50%, 50 mL IV push.
   -Lorazepam (Ativan) 0.1 mg/kg IV at 2 mg/min; may repeat x 1 if seizures continue.

Wernicke-Korsakoff Syndrome:
   -Thiamine 100 mg IV stat, then 100 mg IV qd.

10. **Symptomatic Medications:**
   -Multivitamin 1 amp IV, then 1 tab PO qd.
   -Folate 1 mg PO qd.
   -Thiamine 100 mg PO qd.
   -Acetaminophen (Tylenol) 1-2 PO q4-6h prn headache.
11. **Extras:** CXR, ECG. Alcohol rehabilitation and social work consult.
12. **Labs:** CBC, SMA 7&12, Mg, amylase, lipase, liver panel, urine drug screen. UA, INR/PTT.

Toxicology

Poisoning and Drug Overdose

Decontamination:
- **Gastric Lavage:** Place patient left side down, place nasogastric tube, and check position by injecting air and auscultating. Lavage with normal saline until clear fluid, then leave activated charcoal or other antidote. Gastric lavage is contraindicated for corrosives.
- **Cathartics:**
  - Magnesium citrate 6% sln 150-300 mL PO
  - Magnesium sulfate 10% solution 150-300 mL PO.
- **Activated Charcoal:** 50 gm PO (first dose should be given using product containing sorbitol). Repeat q2-6h for large ingestions.
- **Hemodialysis** is indicated for isopropanol, methanol, ethylene glycol, severe salicylate intoxication (>100 mg/dL), lithium, or theophylline (if neurotoxicity, seizures, or coma).

Antidotes:
  Narcotic Overdose:
  - Naloxone (Narcan) 0.4 mg IV/ET/IM/SC, may repeat q2min.
  Methanol Ingestion:
  - Ethanol (10% in D5W) 7.5 mL/kg load, then 1.4 mL/kg/hr IV infusion until methanol level <20 mg/dL. Maintain ethanol level of 100-150 mg/100 mL.
  Ethylene Glycol Ingestion:
  - Fomepizole (Antizol) 15 mg/kg IV over 30 min, then 10 mg/kg IV q12h x 4 doses, then 15 mg/kg IV q12h until ethylene glycol level is less than 20 mg/dL **AND**
  - Pyridoxine 100 mg IV q6h for 2 days and thiamine 100 mg IV q6h for 2 days.
  Carbon Monoxide Intoxication:
  - Hyperbaric oxygen therapy or 100% oxygen by mask if hyperbaric oxygen not available.
  Tricyclic Antidepressants Overdose:
  - Gastric lavage
  - Magnesium citrate 300 mg PO/NG x1
  - Activated charcoal premixed with sorbitol 50 gm NG q4-6h until level is less than the toxic range.
  Benzodiazepine Overdose:
  - Flumazenil (Romazicon) 0.2 mg (2 mL) IV over 30 seconds q1min until a total dose of 3 mg; if a partial response occurs, repeat 0.5 mg doses until a total of 5 mg. If sedation persists, repeat the above regimen or start a continuous IV infusion of 0.1-0.5 mg/h.

Labs: Drug screen (serum, gastric, urine); blood levels, SMA 7, fingerstick glucose, CBC, LFTs, ECG.

Acetaminophen Overdose

1. **Admit to:** Medical intensive care unit.
2. **Diagnosis:** Acetaminophen overdose
3. **Condition:**
4. **Vital Signs:** q1h with neurochecks. Call physician if BP >160/90, <90/60; P >130, <50 <50; R>25, <10; urine output <20 cc/h for 3 hours.
5. **Activity:** Bed rest with bedside commode.
6. **Nursing:** Inputs and outputs, aspiration and seizure precautions. Place large bore (Ewald) NG tube, then lavage with 2 L of NS.
7. **Diet:** NPO
8. **IV Fluids:**
9. **Special Medications:**
   -Activated charcoal 30-100 gm doses, remove via NG suction prior to acetylcysteine.
   -Acetylcysteine (Mucomyst, NAC) 5% solution loading dose 140 mg/kg via NG tube, then 70 mg/kg via NG tube q4h x 17 doses **OR** acetylcysteine 150 mg/kg IV in 200 mL D5W over 15 min, followed by 50 mg/kg in 500 mL D5W, infused over 4h, followed by 100 mg/kg in 1000 mL of D5W over next 16h. Complete all NAC doses even if acetaminophen levels fall below toxic range.
   -Phytonadione 5 mg IV/IM/SQ (if INR increased).
   -Fresh frozen plasma 2-4 U (if INR is unresponsive to phytonadione).
   -Trimethobenzamide (Tigan) 100-200 mg IM/PR q6h prn nausea
10. **Extras:** ECG. Nephrology consult for hemodialysis or charcoal hemoperfusion.
11. **Labs:** CBC, SMA 7&12, LFTs, INR/PTT, acetaminophen level now and in 4h. UA.

Theophylline Overdose

1. **Admit to:** Medical intensive care unit.
2. **Diagnosis:** Theophylline overdose
3. **Condition:**
4. **Vital Signs:** Neurochecks q2h. Call physician if BP >160/90, <90/60; P >130; <50; R >25, <10.
5. **Activity:** Bed rest
6. **Nursing:** ECG monitoring until level <20 mcg/mL, aspiration and seizure precautions. Insert single lumen NG tube and lavage with normal saline if recent ingestion.
7. **Diet:** NPO
8. **IV Fluids:** D5 ½ NS at 125 cc/h
9. **Special Medications:**
   -Activated charcoal 50 gm PO q4-6h, with sorbitol cathartic, until theophylline level <20 mcg/mL. Maintain head-of-bed at 30-45 degrees to prevent aspiration of charcoal.
   -Charcoal hemoperfusion is indicated if the serum level is >60 mcg/mL or if signs of neurotoxicity, seizure, coma are present.
   -**Seizure:** Lorazepam (Ativan) 0.1 mg/kg IV at 2 mg/min; may repeat x 1 if seizures continue.

10. Extras: ECG.
11. Labs: CBC, SMA 7&12, theophylline level now and in q6-8h; INR/PTT, liver panel. UA.

Tricyclic Antidepressant Overdose

1. **Admit to:** Medical intensive care unit.
2. **Diagnosis:** TCA Overdose
3. **Condition:**
4. **Vital Signs:** Neurochecks q1h.
5. **Activity:** Bedrest.
6. **Nursing:** Continuous suicide observation. ECG monitoring, measure QRS width hourly, inputs and outputs, aspiration and seizure precautions. Place single-lumen nasogastric tube and lavage with 2 liters of normal saline if recent ingestion.
7. **Diet:** NPO
8. **IV Fluids:** NS at 100-150 cc/hr.
9. **Special Medications:**
   -Activated charcoal premixed with sorbitol 50 gm via NG tube q4-6h until the TCA level decreases to therapeutic range. Maintain head-of-bed at 30-45 degree angle to prevent charcoal aspiration.
   -Magnesium citrate 300 mL via nasogastric tube x 1 dose.
10. **Cardiac Toxicity:**
    -If mechanical ventilation is necessary, hyperventilate to maintain pH 7.50-7.55.
    -Administer sodium bicarbonate 50-100 mEq (1-2 amps or 1-2 mEq/kg) IV over 5-10 min, followed by infusion of sodium bicarbonate (2 amps in D5W 1 L) at 100-150 cc/h. Adjust rate to maintain pH 7.50-7.55.
11. **Extras:** ECG.
12. **Labs:** Urine toxicology screen, serum TCA levels, liver panel, CBC, SMA-7 and 12, UA.

Neurologic Disorders

Ischemic Stroke

1. **Admit to:**
2. **Diagnosis:** Ischemic stroke
3. **Condition:**
4. **Vital Signs:** Vital signs and neurochecks q30minutes for 6 hours, then q60 minutes for 12 hours. Call physician if BP >185/105, <110/60; P >120, <50; R>24, <10; T >38.5°C; or change in neurologic status.
5. **Activity:** Bedrest.
6. **Nursing:** Head-of-bed at 30 degrees, turn q2h when awake, range of motion exercises qid. Foley catheter, eggcrate mattress. Guaiac stools, inputs and outputs's.
   Bleeding precautions: check puncture sites for bleeding or hematomas. Apply digital pressure or pressure dressing to active compressible bleeding sites.
7. **Diet:** NPO except medications for 24 hours, then dysphagia ground diet with thickened liquids.
8. **IV Fluids and Oxygen:** 0.45% normal saline at 100 cc/h. Oxygen at 2 L per minute by nasal cannula.
9. **Special Medications:**
Ischemic Stroke < 3 hours:
   a. Tissue plasminogen activator (t-PA, Alteplase) is indicated if the patient presents within 3 hours of onset of symptoms and the stroke is non-hemorrhagic; 0.9 mg/kg (max 90 mg) over 60 min, with 10% of the total dose given as an initial bolus over 1 minute.
   b. Repeat CT scan or MRI 24 hours after completion of tPA. Begin heparin if results of scan are negative for hemorrhage.
   c. Heparin 12 U/kg/h continuous IV infusion, without a bolus. Check aPTT q6h to maintain 1.2-1.5 x control.
Completed Ischemic Stroke >3 hours:
   -Aspirin enteric coated 325 mg PO qd **OR**
   -Clopidogrel (Plavix) 75 mg PO qd **OR**
   -Aspirin 25 mg/dipyridamole 200 mg (Aggrenox) 1 tab PO bid.
10. **Symptomatic Medications:**
   -Famotidine (Pepcid) 20 mg IV/PO q12h.
   -Omeprazole (Prilosec) 20 mg PO bid or qhs.
   -Docusate sodium (Colace) 100 mg PO qhs
   -Bisacodyl (Dulcolax) 10-15 mg PO qhs or 10 mg PR prn.
   -Acetaminophen (Tylenol) 650 mg PO/PR q4-6h prn temp >38°C or headache.
11. **Extras:** CXR, ECG, CT without contrast or MRI with gadolinium contrast; carotid duplex scan; echocardiogram, 24-hour Holter monitor; swallowing studies. Physical therapy consult for range of motion exercises; neurology, rehabilitation medicine consults.
12. **Labs:** CBC, glucose, SMA 7&12, fasting lipid profile, VDRL, ESR; drug levels, INR/PTT, UA. Lupus anticoagulant, anticardiolipin antibody.

Transient Ischemic Attack

1. **Admit to:**
2. **Diagnosis:** Transient ischemic attack
3. **Condition:**
4. **Vital Signs:** q1h with neurochecks. Call physician if BP >160/90, <90/60; P >120, <50; R>25, <10; T >38.5°C; or change in neurologic status.
5. **Activity:** Up as tolerated.
6. **Nursing:** Guaiac stools.
7. **Diet:** Dysphagia ground with thickened liquids or regular diet.
8. **IV Fluids:** Heparin lock with flush q shift.
9. **Special Medications:**
   -Aspirin 325 mg PO qd **OR**
   -Clopidogrel (Plavix) 75 mg PO qd **OR**
   -Aspirin 25 mg/dipyridamole 200 mg (Aggrenox) 1 tab PO bid.
   -Heparin (only if recurrent TIAs or cardiogenic or vertebrobasilar source for emboli) 700-800 U/h (12 U/kg/h) IV infusion without a bolus (25,000 U in 500 mL D5W); adjust q6-12h until PTT 1.2-1.5 x control.
   -Warfarin (Coumadin) 5.0-7.5 mg PO qd for 3d, then 2-4 mg PO qd. Titrate to INR of 2.0-2.5.
10. **Symptomatic Medications:**
    -Famotidine (Pepcid) 20 mg IV/PO q12h.
    -Docusate sodium (Colace) 100 mg PO qhs.
    -Milk of magnesia 30 mL PO qd prn constipation.
11. **Extras:** CXR, ECG, CT without contrast; carotid duplex scan, echocardiogram, 24-hour Holter monitor. Physical therapy, neurology consults.
12. **Labs:** CBC, glucose, SMA 7&12, fasting lipid profile, VDRL, drug levels, INR/PTT, UA.

Subarachnoid Hemorrhage

1. **Admit to:**
2. **Diagnosis:** Subarachnoid hemorrhage
3. **Condition:**
4. **Vital Signs:** Vital signs and neurochecks q1-6h. Call physician if BP >185/105, <110/60; P >120, <50; R>24, <10; T >38.5°C; or change in neurologic status.
5. **Activity:** Bedrest.
6. **Nursing:** Head-of-bed at 30 degrees, turn q2h when awake. Foley catheter, eggcrate mattress. Guaiac stools, inputs and outputs's.
   Bleeding precautions: check puncture sites for bleeding or hematomas. Apply digital pressure or pressure dressing to active compressible bleeding sites.
7. **Diet:** NPO except medications.
8. **IV Fluids and Oxygen:** 0.45% normal saline at 100 cc/h. Oxygen at 2 L per minute by nasal cannula.
   -Keep room dark and quiet; strict bedrest. Neurologic checks q1h for 12 hours, then q2h for 12 hours, then q4h. Call physician if abrupt change in neurologic status.
   -Restrict total fluids to 1000 mL/day; diet as tolerated.

9. Special Medications:
  -Nimodipine (Nimotop) 60 mg PO or via NG tube q4h for 21d, must start within 96 hours.
  -Phenytoin (seizures) load 15 mg/kg IV in NS (infuse at max 50 mg/min), then 300 mg PO/IV qAM (4-6 mg/kg/d).
Hypertension:
  -Nitroprusside sodium, 0.1-0.5 mcg/kg/min (50 mg in 250 mL NS), titrate to control blood pressure.
10. Extras: CXR, ECG, CT without contrast; MRI angiogram; cerebral angiogram. Neurology, neurosurgery consults.
11. Labs: CBC, SMA 7&12, VDRL, UA.

Seizure and Status Epilepticus

1. Admit to:
2. Diagnosis: Seizure
3. Condition:
4. Vital Signs: q6h with neurochecks. Call physician if BP >160/90, <90/60; P >120, <50; R>25, <10; T >38.5°C; or any change in neurological status.
5. Activity: Bed rest
6. Nursing: Finger stick glucose. Seizure precautions with bed rails up; padded tongue blade at bedside. EEG monitoring.
7. Diet: NPO for 24h, then regular diet if alert.
8. IV Fluids: D5 ½ NS at 100 cc/hr; change to heparin lock when taking PO.
9. Special Medications:
Status Epilepticus:
   1. Maintain airway.
   2. Position the patient laterally with the head down. The head and extremities should be cushioned to prevent injury.
   3. A bite block or other soft object may be inserted into the mouth to prevent injury to the tongue.
   4. 100% O_2 by mask, obtain brief history, and a fingerstick glucose.
   5. Secure IV access and draw blood for glucose analysis. Give thiamine 100 mg IV push, then dextrose 50% 50 mL IV push.
   6. **Initial Control:**
      Lorazepam (Ativan) 6-8 mg (0.1 mg/kg; not to exceed 2 mg/min) IV at 1-2 mg/min. May repeat 6-8 mg q5-10min (max 80 mg/24h) **OR**
      Diazepam (Valium), 5-10 mg slow IV at 1-2 mg/min. Repeat 5-10 mg q5-10 min prn (max 100 mg/24h).
      Phenytoin (Dilantin) 15-20 mg/kg load in NS at 50 mg/min. Repeat 100-150 mg IV q30min, max 1.5 gm; monitor BP.
      Fosphenytoin (Cerebyx) 20 mg/kg IV/IM (at 150 mg/min), then 4-6 mg/kg/day in 2 or 3 doses (150 mg IV/IM q8h). Fosphenytoin is metabolized to phenytoin; fosphenytoin may be given IM.
      If Seizures Persist, Administer Phenobarbital 20 mg/kg IV at 50 mg/min, repeat 2 mg/kg q15min; additional phenobarbital may be given, up to max of 30-60 mg/kg.
   7. **If Seizures Persist, Intubate the Patient and Give:**
      - Midazolam (Versed) 0.2 mg/kg IV push, then 0.045 mg/kg/hr; titrate up to 0.6 mg/kg/hr **OR**
      -Propofol (Diprivan) 2 mg/kg IV push, then 2 mg/kg/hr; titrate up to 10

mg/kg/hr **OR**
-Phenobarbital as above.
-Induction of coma with pentobarbital 10-15 mg/kg IV over 1-2h, then 1-1.5 mg/kg/h continuous infusion. Initiate continuous EEG monitoring.

8. Consider Intubation and General Anesthesia

Maintenance Therapy for Epilepsy:

Primary Generalized Seizures – First-Line Therapy:
-Carbamazepine (Tegretol) 200-400 mg PO tid [100, 200 mg]. Monitor CBC.
-Phenytoin (Dilantin) loading dose of 400 mg PO followed by 300 mg PO q4h for 2 doses (total of 1 g), then 300 mg PO qd or 100 mg tid or 200 mg bid [30, 50, 100 mg].
-Divalproex (Depakote) 250-500 mg PO tid-qid with meals [125, 250, 500 mg].
-Valproic acid (Depakene) 250-500 mg PO tid-qid with meals [250 mg].

Primary Generalized Seizures -- Second Line Therapy:
-Phenobarbital 30-120 mg PO bid [8, 16, 32, 65, 100 mg].
-Primidone (Mysoline) 250-500 mg PO tid [50, 250 mg]; metabolized to phenobarbital.
-Felbamate (Felbatol) 1200-2400 mg PO qd in 3-4 divided doses, max 3600 mg/d [400, 600 mg; 600 mg/5 mL susp]; adjunct therapy; aplastic anemia, hepatotoxicity.
-Gabapentin (Neurontin), 300-400 mg PO bid-tid; max 1800 mg/day [100, 300, 400 mg]; adjunct therapy.
-Lamotrigine (Lamictal) 50 mg PO qd, then increase to 50-250 mg PO bid [25, 100, 150, 200 mg]; adjunct therapy .

Partial Seizure:
-Carbamazepine (Tegretol) 200-400 mg PO tid [100, 200 mg].
-Divalproex (Depakote) 250-500 mg PO tid with meals [125, 250, 500 mg].
-Valproic acid (Depakene) 250-500 mg PO tid-qid with meals [250 mg].
-Phenytoin (Dilantin) 300 mg PO qd or 200 mg PO bid [30, 50, 100].
-Phenobarbital 30-120 mg PO tid or qd [8, 16, 32, 65, 100 mg].
-Primidone (Mysoline) 250-500 mg PO tid [50, 250 mg]; metabolized to phenobarbital.
-Felbamate (Felbatol) 1200-2400 mg PO qd in 3-4 divided doses, max 3600 mg/d [400,600 mg; 600 mg/5 mL susp]; adjunct therapy; aplastic anemia, hepatotoxicity.
-Gabapentin (Neurontin), 300-400 mg PO bid-tid; max 1800 mg/day [100, 300, 400 mg]; adjunct therapy.
-Lamotrigine (Lamictal) 50 mg PO qd, then increase to 50-250 mg PO bid [25, 100, 150, 200 mg]; adjunct therapy.
-Topiramate (Topamax) 25 mg PO bid; titrate to max 200 mg PO bid [tab 25, 100, 200 mg]; adjunctive therapy.

Absence Seizure:
-Divalproex (Depakote) 250-500 mg PO tid-qid [125, 250, 500 mg].
-Clonazepam (Klonopin) 0.5-5 mg PO bid-qid [0.5, 1, 2 mg].
-Lamotrigine (Lamictal) 50 mg PO qd, then increase to 50-250 mg PO bid [25, 100, 150, 200 mg]; adjunct therapy.

10. Extras: MRI with and without gadolinium or CT with contrast; EEG (with photic stimulation, hyperventilation, sleep deprivation, awake and asleep tracings); portable CXR, ECG.

11. Labs: CBC, SMA 7, glucose, Mg, calcium, phosphate, liver panel, VDRL, anticonvulsant levels. UA, drug screen.

Endocrinologic Disorders

Diabetic Ketoacidosis

1. **Admit to:**
2. **Diagnosis:** Diabetic ketoacidosis
3. **Condition:**
4. **Vital Signs:** q1-4h, postural BP and pulse. Call physician if BP >160/90, <90/60; P >140, <50; R >30, <10; T >38.5°C; or urine output < 20 mL/hr for more than 2 hours.
5. **Activity:** Bed rest with bedside commode.
6. **Nursing:** Inputs and outputs. Foley to closed drainage. Record labs on flow sheet.
7. **Diet:** NPO for 12 hours, then clear liquids as tolerated.
8. **IV Fluids:**
   1-2 L NS over 1-3h (≥16 gauge), infuse at 400-1000 mL/h until hemodynamically stable, then change to 0.45% saline at 125-150 cc/hr; keep urine output >30-60 mL/h.
   Add KCL when serum potassium is <5.0 mEq/L.
       Concentration.......20-40 mEq KCL/L
   May use K phosphate, 20-40 mEq/L, in place of KCL if hypophosphatemic.
   Change to 5% dextrose in 0.45% saline with 20-40 mEq KCL/liter when blood glucose 250-300 mg/dL.
9. **Special Medications:**
   -Oxygen at 2 L/min by NC.
   -Insulin regular (Humulin) 7-10 units (0.1 U/kg) IV bolus, then 7-10 U/h IV infusion (0.1 U/kg/h); 50 U in 250 mL of 0.9% saline; flush IV tubing with 20 mL of insulin sln before starting infusion. Adjust insulin infusion to decrease serum glucose by 100 mg/dL or less per hour. When bicarbonate level is >16 mEq/L and anion gap is <16 mEq/L, decrease insulin infusion rate by half.
   -When the glucose level reaches 250 mg/dL, 5% dextrose should be added to the replacement fluids with KCL 20-40 mEq/L.
   -Use 10% glucose at 50-100 mL/h if anion gap persists and serum glucose has decreased to less than 100 mg/dL while on insulin infusion.
   -Change to subcutaneous insulin when anion gap cleared; discontinue insulin infusion 1-2h after subcutaneous dose.
10. **Symptomatic Medications:**
    -Docusate sodium (Colace) 100 mg PO qhs.
    -Acetaminophen (Tylenol) 325-650 mg PO q4-6h prn headache.
11. **Extras:** Portable CXR, ECG.
12. **Labs:** Fingerstick glucose q1-2h. SMA 7 q4-6h. SMA 12, pH, bicarbonate, phosphate, amylase, lipase, hemoglobin A1c; CBC. UA, serum pregnancy test.

Nonketotic Hyperosmolar Syndrome

1. **Admit to:**
2. **Diagnosis:** Nonketotic hyperosmolar syndrome
3. **Condition:**
4. **Vital Signs:** q1h. Call physician if BP >160/90, <90/60; P >140, <50; R>25, <10; T >38.5° C; or urine output <20 cc/hr for more than 4 hours.
5. **Activity:** Bed rest with bedside commode.
6. **Nursing:** Input and output measurement. Foley to closed drainage. Record labs on flow sheet.
7. **Diet:** NPO.
8. **IV Fluids:** 1-2 L NS over 1h (≥16 gauge IV catheter), then give 0.45% saline at 125 cc/hr. Maintain urine output ≥50 mL/h.
   -Add 20-40 mEq/L KCL when urine output adequate.
9. **Special Medications:**
   -Insulin regular 2-3 U/h IV infusion (50 U in 250 mL of 0.9% saline).
   -Famotidine (Pepcid) 20 mg IV/PO q12h.
   -Heparin 5000 U SQ q12h.
10. **Extras:** Portable CXR, ECG.
11. **Labs:** Fingerstick glucose q1-2h x 6h, then q6h. SMA 7, osmolality. SMA 12, phosphate, ketones, hemoglobin A1C, CBC. UA.

Thyroid Storm and Hyperthyroidism

1. **Admit to:**
2. **Diagnosis:** Thyroid Storm
3. **Condition:**
4. **Vital Signs:** q1-4h. Call physician if BP >160/90, <90/60; P >130, <50; R>25, <10; T >38.5°C
5. **Activity:** Bed rest
6. **Nursing:** Cooling blanket prn temp >39°C, inputs and outputs. Oxygen 2 L/min by nasal canula.
7. **Diet:** Regular
8. **IV Fluids:** D5 ½ NS at 125 mL/h.
9. **Special Medications:**
Thyroid Storm and Hyperthyroidism:
   -Methimazole (Tapazole) 30-60 mg PO, then maintenance of 15 mg PO qd-bid **OR**
   -Propylthiouracil (PTU) 1000 mg PO, then 50-250 mg PO q4-8h, up to 1200 mg/d; usual maintenance dose 50 mg PO tid **AND**
   -Iodide solution (Lugol's solution), 3-6 drops tid; one hour after propylthiouracil **AND**
   -Dexamethasone (Decadron) 2 mg IV q6h **AND**
   -Propranolol 40-160 mg PO q6h or 5-10 mg/h, max 2-5 mg IV q4h or propranolol-LA (Inderal-LA), 80-120 mg PO qd [60, 80, 120, 160 mg].
   -Acetaminophen (Tylenol) 1-2 tabs PO q4-6h prn temp >38°C.
   -Zolpidem (Ambien) 10 mg PO qhs prn insomnia **OR**
   -Lorazepam (Ativan) 1-2 mg IV/IM/PO q4-8h prn anxiety.
10. **Extras:** CXR PA and LAT, ECG, endocrine consult.
11. **Labs:** CBC, SMA 7&12; sensitive TSH, free T4. UA.

Myxedema Coma and Hypothyroidism

1. **Admit to:**
2. **Diagnosis:** Myxedema Coma
3. **Condition:**
4. **Vital Signs:** q1h. Call physician if BP systolic >160/90, <90/60; P >130, <50; R>25, <10; T >38.5°C
5. **Activity:** Bed rest
6. **Nursing:** Triple blankets prn temp <36°C, inputs and outputs, aspiration precautions.
7. **Diet:** NPO
8. **IV Fluids:** IV D5 NS TKO.
9. **Special Medications:**

Myxedema Coma and Hypothyroidism:
   -Volume replacement with NS 1 L rapid IV, then 125 mL/h.
   -Levothyroxine (Synthroid, Levoxine) 300-500 mcg IV, then 100 mcg PO or IV qd.
   -Hydrocortisone 100 mg IV loading dose, then 50-100 mg IV q8h.

Hypothyroidism in Medically Stable Patient:
   -Levothyroxine (Synthroid, T4) 50-75 mcg PO qd, increase by 25 mcg PO qd at 2-4 week intervals to 75-150 mcg qd until TSH normalized.

11. **Extras:** ECG, endocrine consult.
12. **Labs:** CBC, SMA 7&12; sensitive TSH, free T4. UA, rheumatoid factor, ANA.

Nephrologic Disorders

Renal Failure

1. **Admit to:**
2. **Diagnosis:** Renal failure
3. **Condition:**
4. **Vital Signs:** q8h. Call physician if QRS complex >0.14 sec; urine output <20 cc/hr; BP >160/90, <90/60; P >120, <50; R>25, <10; T >38.5°C
5. **Allergies:** Avoid magnesium containing antacids, salt substitutes, NSAIDS. Discontinue phosphate or potassium supplements.
6. **Activity:** Bed rest.
7. **Nursing:** Daily weights, inputs and outputs, chart urine output. If no urine output for 4h, in-and-out catheterize. Guaiac stools.
8. **Diet:** Renal diet of high biologic value protein of 0.6-0.8 g/kg, sodium 2 g, potassium 1 mEq/kg, and at least 35 kcal/kg of nonprotein calories. In oliguric patients, daily fluid intake should be restricted to less than 1 L after volume has been normalized.
9. **IV Fluids:** D5W at TKO.
10. **Special Medications:**
    - Consider fluid challenge (to rule out pre-renal azotemia if not fluid overloaded) with 500-1000 mL NS IV over 30 min. In acute renal failure, in-and-out catheterize and check postvoid residual to rule out obstruction.
    - Furosemide (Lasix) 80-320 mg IV bolus over 10-60 min, double the dose if no response after 2 hours to total max 1000 mg/24h, or furosemide 1000 mg in 250 mL D5W at 20-40 mg/hr continuous IV infusion **OR**
    - Torsemide (Demadex) 20-40 mg IV bolus over 5-10 min, double the dose up to max 200 mg/day **OR**
    - Bumetanide (Bumex) 1-2 mg IV bolus over 1-20 min; double the dose if no response in 1-2 h to total max 10 mg/day.
    - Metolazone (Zaroxolyn) 5-10 mg PO (max 20 mg/24h) 30 min before a loop diuretic.
    - Dopamine (Intropin) 1-3 mcg/kg per minute IV.
    - Hyperkalemia is treated with sodium polystyrene sulfonate (Kayexalate), 15-30 gm PO/NG/PR q4-6h.
    - Hyperphosphatemia is controlled with calcium acetate (PhosLo), 2-3 tabs with meals.
    - Metabolic acidosis is treated with sodium bicarbonate to maintain the serum pH >7.2 and the bicarbonate level >20 mEq/L. 1-2 amps (50-100 mEq) IV push, followed by infusion of 2-3 amps in 1000 mL of D5W at 150 mL/hr.
    - Adjust all medications to creatinine clearance, and remove potassium phosphate and magnesium from IV. Avoid NSAIDs and nephrotoxic drugs.
11. **Extras:** CXR, ECG, renal ultrasound, nephrology and dietetics consults.
12. **Labs:** CBC, platelets, SMA 7&12, creatinine, BUN, potassium, magnesium, phosphate, calcium, uric acid, osmolality, ESR, INR/PTT, ANA. Urine specific gravity, UA with micro, urine C&S; 1st AM spot urine electrolytes, eosinophils, creatinine, pH, osmolality; Wright's stain, urine electrophoresis. 24h urine protein, creatinine, sodium.

Nephrolithiasis

1. **Admit to:**
2. **Diagnosis:** Nephrolithiasis
3. **Condition:**
4. **Vital Signs:** q8h. Call physician if urine output <30 cc/hr; BP >160/90, <90/60; T >38.5°C
5. **Activity:** Up ad lib.
6. **Nursing:** Strain urine, measure inputs and outputs. Place Foley if no urine for 4 hours.
7. **Diet:** Regular, push oral fluids.
8. **IV Fluids:** IV D5 ½ NS at 100-125 cc/hr (maintain urine output of 80 mL/h).
9. **Special Medications:**
   -Cefazolin (Ancef) 1-2 gm IV q8h
   -Meperidine (Demerol) 75-100 mg and hydroxyzine 25 mg IM/IV q2-4h prn pain **OR**
   -Butorphanol (Stadol) 0.5-2 mg IV q3-4h.
   -Hydrocodone/acetaminophen (Vicodin), 1-2 tab q4-6h PO prn pain **OR**
   -Oxycodone/acetaminophen (Percocet) 1 tab q6h prn pain **OR**
   -Acetaminophen with codeine (Tylenol 3) 1-2 tabs PO q3-4h prn pain.
   -Ketorolac (Toradol) 10 mg PO q4-6h prn pain, or 30-60 mg IV/IM then 15-30 mg IV/IM q6h (max 5 days).
   -Zolpidem (Ambien) 10 mg PO qhs prn insomnia.
11. **Extras:** Intravenous pyelogram, KUB, CXR, ECG.
12. **Labs:** CBC, SMA 6 and 12, calcium, uric acid, phosphorous, UA with micro, urine C&S, urine pH, INR/PTT. Urine cystine (nitroprusside test), send stones for X-ray crystallography. 24 hour urine collection for uric acid, calcium, creatinine.

Hypercalcemia

1. **Admit to:**
2. **Diagnosis:** Hypercalcemia
3. **Condition:**
4. **Vital Signs:** q4h. Call physician if BP >160/90, <90/60; P >120, <50; R>25, <10; T >38.5°C; or tetany or any abnormal mental status.
5. **Activity:** Encourage ambulation; up in chair at other times.
6. **Nursing:** Seizure precautions, measure inputs and outputs.
7. **Diet:** Restrict dietary calcium to 400 mg/d, push PO fluids.
8. **Special Medications:**
   -1-2 L of 0.9% saline over 1-4 hours until no longer hypotensive, then saline diuresis with 0.9% saline infused at 125 cc/h **AND**
   -Furosemide (Lasix) 20-80 mg IV q4-12h. Maintain urine output of 200 mL/h; monitor serum sodium, potassium, magnesium.
   -Calcitonin (Calcimar) 4-8 IV kg IM q12h or SQ q6-12h.
   -Etidronate (Didronel) 7.5 mg/kg/day in 250 mL of normal saline IV infusion over 2 hours. Repeat on 3 days.
   -Pamidronate (Aredia) 60 mg in 1 liter of NS infused over 4 hours or 90 mg in 1 liter of NS infused over 24 hours x one dose.
9. **Extras:** CXR, ECG, mammogram.
10. **Labs:** Total and ionized calcium, parathyroid hormone, SMA 7&12, phos-

phate, Mg, alkaline phosphatase, prostate specific antigen and carcinoembryonic antigen. 24h urine calcium, phosphate.

Hypocalcemia

1. **Admit to:**
2. **Diagnosis:** Hypocalcemia
3. **Condition:**
4. **Vital Signs:** q4h. Call physician if BP >160/90, <90/60; P >120, <50; R>25, <10; T >38.5°C; or any abnormal mental status.
5. **Activity:** Up ad lib
6. **Nursing:** I and O.
7. **Diet:** No added salt diet.
8. **Special Medications:**

Symptomatic Hypocalcemia:
-Calcium chloride, 10% (270 mg calcium/10 mL vial) give 5-10 mL slowly over 10 min or dilute in 50-100 mL of D5W and infuse over 20 min, repeat q20-30 min if symptomatic, or hourly if asymptomatic. Correct hyperphosphatemia before hypocalcemia **OR**
-Calcium gluconate, 20 mL of 10% solution IV (2 vials)(90 mg elemental calcium/10 mL vial) infused over 10-15 min, followed by infusion of 60 mL of calcium gluconate in 500 cc of D5W (1 mg/mL) at 0.5-2.0 mg/kg/h.

Chronic Hypocalcemia:
-Calcium carbonate with vitamin D (Oscal-D) 1-2 tab PO tid **OR**
-Calcium carbonate (Oscal) 1-2 tab PO tid **OR**
-Calcium citrate (Citracal) 1 tab PO q8h or Extra strength Tums 1-2 PO with meals.
-Vitamin D2 (Ergocalciferol) 1 tab PO qd.
-Calcitriol (Rocaltrol) 0.25 mcg PO qd, titrate up to 0.5-2.0 mcg qid.
-Docusate sodium (Colace) 1 tab PO bid.

9. **Extras:** CXR, ECG.
10. **Labs:** SMA 7&12, phosphate, Mg. 24h urine calcium, potassium, phosphate, magnesium.

Hyperkalemia

1. **Admit to:**
2. **Diagnosis:** Hyperkalemia
3. **Condition:**
4. **Vital Signs:** q4h. Call physician if QRS complex >0.14 sec or BP >160/90, <90/60; P >120, <50; R>25, <10; T >38.5°C.
5. **Activity:** Bed rest; up in chair as tolerated.
6. **Nursing:** Inputs and outputs. Chart QRS complex width q1h.
7. **Diet:** Regular, no salt substitutes.
8. **IV Fluids:** D5NS at 125 cc/h
9. **Special Medications:**
    -Consider discontinuing ACE inhibitors, angiotensin II receptor blockers, beta-blockers, potassium sparing diuretics.
    -Calcium gluconate (10% sln) 10-30 mL IV over 2-5 min; second dose may

    be given in 5 min. Contraindicated if digoxin toxicity is suspected. Keep 10 mL vial of calcium gluconate at bedside for emergent use.

-Sodium bicarbonate 1 amp (50 mEq) IV over 5 min (give after calcium in separate IV).

-Regular insulin 10 units IV push with 1 ampule of 50% glucose IV push.

-Kayexalate 30-45 gm premixed in sorbitol solution PO/NG/PR now and in q3-4h prn.

-Furosemide 40-80 mg IV, repeat prn.

-Consider emergent dialysis if cardiac complications or renal failure.

10. Extras: ECG.

11. Labs: CBC, platelets, SMA7, magnesium, calcium, SMA-12. UA, urine specific gravity, urine sodium, pH, 24h urine potassium, creatinine.

Hypokalemia

1. Admit to:

2. Diagnosis: Hypokalemia

3. Condition:

4. Vital Signs: Vitals, urine output q4h. Call physician if BP >160/90, <90/60; P>120, <50; R>25, <10; T >38.5°C.

5. Activity: Bed rest; up in chair as tolerated.

6. Nursing: Inputs and outputs

7. Diet: Regular

8. Special Medications:

Acute Therapy:

    -KCL 20-40 mEq in 100 cc saline infused IVPB over 2 hours; or add 40-80 mEq to 1 liter of IV fluid and infuse over 4-8 hours.

    -KCL elixir 40 mEq PO tid (in addition to IV); max total dose 100-200 mEq/d (3 mEq/kg/d).

Chronic Therapy:

    -Micro-K 10 mEq tabs 2-3 tabs PO tid after meals (40-100 mEq/d) **OR**

    -K-Dur 20 mEq tabs 1 PO bid-tid.

Hypokalemia with metabolic acidosis:

    -Potassium citrate 15-30 mL in juice PO qid after meals (1 mEq/mL).

    -Potassium gluconate 15 mL in juice PO qid after meals (20 mEq/15 mL).

9. Extras: ECG, dietetics consult.

10. Labs: CBC, magnesium, SMA 7&12. UA, urine Na, pH, 24h urine for K, creatinine.

Hypermagnesemia

1. Admit to:

2. Diagnosis: Hypermagnesemia

3. Condition:

4. Vital Signs: q6h. Call physician if QRS >0.14 sec.

5. Activity: Up ad lib

6. Nursing: Inputs and outputs, daily weights.

7. Diet: Regular

8. **Special Medications:**
   -Saline diuresis 0.9% saline infused at 100-200 cc/h to replace urine loss **AND**
   -Calcium chloride, 1-3 gm added to saline (10% sln; 1 gm per 10 mL amp) to run at 1 gm/hr **AND**
   -Furosemide (Lasix) 20-40 mg IV q4-6h as needed.
   -Magnesium of >9.0 requires stat hemodialysis because of risk of respiratory failure.

9. **Extras:** ECG

10. **Labs:** Magnesium, calcium, SMA 7&12, creatinine. 24 hour urine magnesium, creatinine.

Hypomagnesemia

1. **Admit to:**
2. **Diagnosis:** Hypomagnesemia
3. **Condition:**
4. **Vital Signs:** q6h
5. **Activity:** Up ad lib
6. **Diet:** Regular
7. **Special Medications:**
   -Magnesium sulfate 4-6 gm in 500 mL D5W IV at 1 gm/hr. Hold if no patellar reflex. (Estimation of Mg deficit = 0.2 x kg weight x desired increase in Mg concentration; give deficit over 2-3d) **OR**
   -Magnesium sulfate (severe hypomagnesemia <1.0) 1-2 gm (2-4 mL of 50% sln) IV over 15 min, **OR**
   -Magnesium chloride (Slow-Mag) 65-130 mg (1-2 tabs) PO tid-qid (64 mg or 5.3 mEq/tab) **OR**
   -Milk of magnesia 5 mL PO qd-qid.

8. **Extras:** ECG

9. **Labs:** Magnesium, calcium, SMA 7&12. Urine Mg, electrolytes, 24h urine magnesium, creatinine.

Hypernatremia

1. **Admit to:**
2. **Diagnosis:** Hypernatremia
3. **Condition:**
4. **Vital Signs:** q2-8h. Call physician if BP >160/90, <70/50; P >140, <50; R>25, <10; T >38.5°C.
5. **Activity:** Bed rest; up in chair as tolerated.
6. **Nursing:** Inputs and outputs, daily weights.
7. **Diet:** No added salt.
8. **Special Medications:**
Hypernatremia with Hypovolemia:
   If volume depleted, give 1-2 L NS IV over 1-3 hours until not orthostatic, then give D5W IV or PO to replace half of body water deficit over first 24hours

(attempt to correct sodium at 1 mEq/L/h), then remaining deficit over
next 1-2 days.

Body water deficit (L) = $\dfrac{0.6(\text{weight kg})([\text{Na serum}]-140)}{140}$

Hypernatremia with ECF Volume Excess:
    -Furosemide 40-80 mg IV or PO qd-bid.
    -Salt poor albumin (25%) 50-100 mL bid-tid x 48-72 h.

Hypernatremia with Diabetes Insipidus:
    -D5W to correct body water deficit (see above).
    -Pitressin 5-10 U IM/IV q6h or desmopressin (DDAVP) 4 mcg IV/SQ q12h;
        keep urine specific gravity >1.010.

9. Extras: CXR, ECG.
10. Labs: SMA 7&12, serum osmolality, liver panel, ADH, plasma renin activity.
UA, urine specific gravity. Urine osmolality, Na, 24h urine K, creatinine.

Hyponatremia

1. Admit to:
2. Diagnosis: Hyponatremia
3. Condition:
4. Vital Signs: q4h. Call physician if BP >160/90, <70/50; P >140, <50; R>25,
    <10; T >38.5°C.
5. Activity: Up in chair as tolerated.
6. Nursing: Inputs and outputs, daily weights.
7. Diet: Regular diet.
8. Special Medications:
**Hyponatremia with Hypervolemia and Edema (low osmolality <280, UNa
<10 mmol/L: nephrosis, heart failure, cirrhosis):**
    -Water restrict to 0.5-1.0 L/d.
    -Furosemide 40-80 mg IV or PO qd-bid.

**Hyponatremia with Normal Volume Status (low osmolality <280, UNa <10
mmol: water intoxication; UNa >20: SIADH, diuretic-induced):**
    -Water restrict to 0.5-1.5 L/d.

Hyponatremia with Hypovolemia (low osmolality <280) UNa <10 mmol/L:
vomiting, diarrhea, third space/respiratory/skin loss; UNa >20 mmol/L: diuretics,
renal injury, RTA, adrenal insufficiency, partial obstruction, salt wasting:
    -If volume depleted, give 0.5-2 L of 0.9% saline over 1-2 hours until no longer
        hypotensive, then 0.9% saline at 125 mL/h or 100-500 mL 3% hypertonic
        saline over 4h.

Severe Symptomatic Hyponatremia:
    If volume depleted, give 1-2 L of 0.9% saline (154 mEq/L) over 1-2 hours until
    no longer orthostatic.
    Determine volume of 3% hypertonic saline (513 mEq/L) to be infused:

Na (mEq) deficit = 0.6 x (wt kg)x(desired [Na] - actual [Na])

$$\frac{\text{Volume of sln (L)}}{\text{Number of hrs}} = \frac{\text{Sodium to be infused (mEq)}}{\text{(mEq/L in sln) x Number of hrs}}$$

-Correct half of sodium deficit intravenously over 24 hours until serum sodium
is 120 mEq/L; increase sodium by 12-20 mEq/L over 24 hours (1 mEq/L/h).
-Alternative Method: 3% saline 100-300 mL over 4-6h, repeated as needed.
9. Extras: CXR, ECG, head/chest CT scan.
10. Labs: SMA 7&12, osmolality, triglyceride, liver panel. UA, urine specific
gravity. Urine osmolality, Na.

Hyperphosphatemia

1. Admit to:
2. Diagnosis: Hyperphosphatemia
3. Condition:
4. Vital Signs: qid
5. Activity: Up ad lib
6. Nursing: Inputs and outputs
7. Diet: Low phosphorus diet with 0.7-1 gm/d
8. Special Medications:
Moderate Hyperphosphatemia:
-Restrict dietary phosphate to 0.7-1.0 gm/d.
-Calcium acetate (PhosLo) 1-3 tabs PO tid with meals, **OR**
-Aluminum hydroxide (Amphojel) 5-10 mL or 1-2 tablets PO before meals tid.
Severe Hyperphosphatemia:
-Volume expansion with 0.9% saline 1-2 L over 1-2h.
-Acetazolamide (Diamox) 500 mg PO or IV q6h.
-Consider dialysis.
9. Extras: CXR PA and LAT, ECG.
10. Labs: Phosphate, SMA 7&12, magnesium, calcium. UA, parathyroid
hormone.

Hypophosphatemia

1. Admit to:
2. Diagnosis: Hypophosphatemia
3. Condition:
4. Vital Signs: qid
5. Activity: Up ad lib
6. Nursing: Inputs and outputs.
7. Diet: Regular diet.
8. Special Medications:
Mild to Moderate Hypophosphatemia (1.0-2.2 mg/dL):
-Sodium or potassium phosphate 0.25 mMoles/kg in 150-250 mL of NS or
D5W at 10 mMoles/h.
-Neutral phosphate (Nutra-Phos), 2 tab PO bid (250 mg elemental phosphorus/tab) **OR**
-Phospho-Soda 5 mL (129 mg phosphorus) PO bid-tid.

Severe Hypophosphatemia (<1.0 mg/dL):
  -Na or K phosphate 0.5 mMoles/kg in 250 mL D5W or NS, IV infusion at 10
    mMoles/hr **OR**
  -Add potassium phosphate to IV solution in place of maintenance KCL; max
    IV dose 7.5 mg phosphorus/kg/6h.
9. **Extras:** CXR PA and LAT, ECG.
10. **Labs:** Phosphate, SMA 7&12, Mg, calcium, UA.

Rheumatologic Disorders

Systemic Lupus Erythematosus

1. **Admit to:**
2. **Diagnosis:** Systemic Lupus Erythematosus
3. **Condition:**
4. **Vital Signs:** tid
5. **Allergies:**
6. **Activity:** Up as tolerated with bathroom privileges
7. **Nursing:**
8. **Diet:** No added salt, low psoralen diet.
9. **Special Medications:**
   -Ibuprofen (Motrin) 400 mg PO qid (max 2.4 g/d) **OR**
   -Indomethacin (Indocin) 25-50 mg tid-qid.
   -Hydroxychloroquine (Plaquenil) 200-600 mg/d PO
   -Prednisone 60-100 mg PO qd, may increase to 200-300 mg/d. Maintenance 10-20 mg PO qd or 20-40 mg PO qOD **OR**
   -Methylprednisolone (pulse therapy) 500 mg IV over 30 min q12h for 3-5d, then prednisone 50 mg PO qd.
   -Betamethasone dipropionate (Diprolene) 0.05% ointment applied bid.
10. **Extras:** CXR PA, LAT, ECG. Rheumatology consult.
11. **Labs:** CBC, platelets, SMA 7&12, INR/PTT, ESR, complement CH-50, C3, C4, C-reactive protein, LE prep, Coombs test, VDRL, rheumatoid factor, ANA, DNA binding, lupus anticoagulant, anticardiolipin, antinuclear cytoplasmic antibody. UA.

Acute Gout Attack

1. **Admit to:**
2. **Diagnosis:** Acute gout attack
3. **Condition:**
4. **Vital Signs:** tid
5. **Activity:** Bed rest with bedside commode
6. **Nursing:** Keep foot elevated; support sheets over foot; guaiac stools.
7. **Diet:** Low purine diet.
8. **Special Medications:**
   -Ibuprofen (Motrin) 800 mg, then 400-800 mg PO q4-6h **OR**
   -Diclofenac (Voltaren) 25-75 mg tid-qid with food **OR**
   -Indomethacin (Indocin) 25-50 mg PO q6h for 2d, then 50 mg tid for 2 days, then 25 mg PO tid **OR**
   -Ketorolac (Toradol) 30-60 mg IV/IM, then 15-30 mg IV/IM q6h or 10 mg PO tid-qid **OR**
   -Naproxen sodium (Anaprox, Anaprox-DS) 550 mg PO bid **OR**
   -Methylprednisolone (SoluMedrol) 125 mg IV x 1 dose **THEN**
   -Prednisone 60 mg PO qd for 5 days, followed by tapering.
   -Colchicine 2 tablets (0.5 mg or 0.6 mg), followed by 1 tablet q1h until relief, max dose of 9.6 mg/24h. Maintenance colchicine: 0.5-0.6 mg PO qd-bid.

Hypouricemic Therapy:
-Probenecid (Benemid), 250 mg bid. Increase the dosage to 500 mg bid after 1 week, then increase by 500-mg increments every 4 weeks until the uric acid level is below 6.5 mg/dL. Max dose 2 g/d. Contraindicated during acute attack.
-Allopurinol (Zyloprim) 300 mg PO qd, may increase by 100-300 mg q2weeks. Usually initiated after the acute attack.

9. **Symptomatic Medications:**
-Famotidine (Pepcid) 20 mg IV/PO q12h.
-Meperidine (Demerol) 50-100 mg IM/IV q4-6h prn pain **OR**
-Hydrocodone/acetaminophen (Vicodin), 1-2 tab q4-6h PO prn pain.
-Docusate sodium (Colace) 100 mg PO qhs.
-Acetaminophen (Tylenol) 325-650 mg PO q4-6h prn headache.
-Zolpidem (Ambien) 5-10 mg qhs prn insomnia.

10. **Labs:** CBC, SMA 7, uric acid. UA with micro. Synovial fluid for light and polarizing micrography for crystals; C&S, Gram stain, glucose, protein, cell count. X-ray views of joint. 24 hour urine for uric acid.

Commonly Used Formulas

A-a gradient = $[(P_B - PH_2O) FiO_2 - PCO_2/R] - PO_2$ arterial

$\qquad$ = $(713 \times FiO_2 - pCO_2/0.8) - pO_2$ arterial

$P_B = 760$ mmHg; $PH_2O = 47$ mmHg ; $R = 0.8$
normal Aa gradient <10-15 mmHg (room air)

Arterial oxygen capacity = (Hgb(gm)/100 mL) x 1.36 mL O_2/gm Hgb

Arterial O_2 content = $1.36(Hgb)(SaO_2) + 0.003(PaO_2)$ = NL 20 vol%

O_2 delivery = CO x arterial O_2 content = NL 640-1000 mL O_2/min

Cardiac output = HR x stroke volume

CO L/min = $\dfrac{125 \text{ mL } O_2/\text{min}/M^2}{8.5\{(1.36)(Hgb)(SaO_2) - (1.36)(Hgb)(SvO_2)\}}$ x 100

Normal CO = 4-6 L/min

Na (mEq) deficit = 0.6 x (wt kg) x (desired [Na] - actual [Na])

SVR = $\dfrac{MAP - CVP}{CO_{L/min}}$ x 80 = NL 800-1200 dyne/sec/cm^2

PVR = $\dfrac{PA - PCWP}{CO_{L/min}}$ x 80 = NL 45-120 dyne/sec/cm^2

GFR mL/min = $\dfrac{(140 - \text{age}) \times \text{ideal weight in kg}}{\substack{72 \text{ (males) x serum creatinine (mg/dL)} \\ 85 \text{ (females) x serum creatinine (mg/dL)}}}$

Creatinine clearance = $\dfrac{U \text{ creatinine (mg/100 mL)} \times U \text{ vol (mL)}}{P \text{ creatinine (mg/100 mL)} \times \text{time (1440 min for 24h)}}$

Normal creatinine clearance = 100-125 mL/min(males), 85-105(females)

Body water deficit (L) = $\dfrac{0.6(\text{weight kg})([\text{measured serum Na}]-140)}{140}$

Serum Osmolality = $2 [Na] + \dfrac{BUN}{2.8} + \dfrac{Glucose}{18}$ = 270-290

Na (mEq) deficit = 0.6 x (wt kg)x(desired [Na] - actual [Na])

Fractional excreted Na = $\dfrac{U \text{ Na/ Serum Na} \times 100}{U \text{ creatinine/ Serum creatinine}}$ = NL<1%

Anion Gap = Na - (Cl + HCO_3)

For each 100 mg/dL increase in glucose, Na decreases by 1.6 mEq/L.

Corrected serum Ca^+ (mg/dL) = measured Ca mg/dL + 0.8 x (4 - albumin g/dL)

Predicted Maximal Heart Rate = 220 - age

Normal ECG Intervals (sec)

PR	0.12-0.20
QRS	0.06-0.08
Heart rate/min	**Q-T**
60	0.33-0.43
70	0.31-0.41
80	0.29-0.38
90	0.28-0.36
100	0.27-0.35

Total Parenteral Nutrition Equations:

Caloric Requirements: (Harris-Benedict Equations)
    Basal energy expenditure (BEE)
        Females: 655 + (9.6 x wt in kg) + (1.85 x ht in cm) - (4.7 x age)
        Males: 66 + (13.7 x wt in kg) + (5 x ht in cm) - (6.8 x age)

    A. BEE x 1.2 = Caloric requirement for minimally stressed patient
    B. BEE x 1.3 = Caloric requirement for moderately stressed patient (inflammatory bowel disease, cancer, surgery)
    C. BEE x 1.5 = Caloric requirement for severely stressed patient (major sepsis, burns, AIDS, liver disease)
    D. BEE x 1.7 = Caloric requirement for extremely stressed patient (traumatic burns >50%, open head trauma, multiple stress)

Protein Requirements:
    A. Protein requirement for non-stressed patient = 0.8 gm protein/kg.
    B. Protein requirement for patients with decreased visceral protein states (hypoalbuminemia), recent weight loss, or hypercatabolic states = 1.0-1.5 gm protein/kg.

Estimation of Ideal Body Weight:
    A. Females: 5 feet (allow 100 lbs) + 5 lbs for each inch over 5 feet
    B. Males: 5 feet (allow 106 lbs) + 6 lbs for each inch over 5 feet

Commonly Used Drug Levels

Drug	Therapeutic Range
Amikacin	Peak 25-30; trough <10 mcg/mL
Amiodarone	1.0-3.0 mcg/mL
Amitriptyline	100-250 ng/mL
Carbamazepine	4-10 mcg/mL
Desipramine	150-300 ng/mL
Digoxin	0.8-2.0 ng/mL
Disopyramide	2-5 mcg/mL
Doxepin	75-200 ng/mL
Flecainide	0.2-1.0 mcg/mL
Gentamicin	Peak 6.0-8.0; trough <2.0 mcg/mL
Imipramine	150-300 ng/mL
Lidocaine	2-5 mcg/mL
Lithium	0.5-1.4 mEq/L
Mexiletine	1.0-2.0 mcg/mL
Nortriptyline	50-150 ng/mL
Phenobarbital	10-30 mEq/mL
Phenytoin	8-20 mcg/mL
Procainamide	4.0-8.0 mcg/mL
Quinidine	2.5-5.0 mcg/mL
Salicylate	15-25 mg/dL
Streptomycin	Peak 10-20; trough <5 mcg/mL
Theophylline	8-20 mcg/mL
Tocainide	4-10 mcg/mL
Valproic acid	50-100 mcg/mL
Vancomycin	Peak 30-40; trough <10 mcg/mL

Extended Interval Gentamicin and Tobramycin Dosing

Estimate the glomerular filtration rate as follows:

Estimated GFR (mL/min) for males $= \dfrac{(140 - \text{age}) \times \text{ideal weight in kg}}{72 \times \text{serum creatinine (mg/dL)}}$

Estimated GFR (mL/min) for females $= \dfrac{(140 - \text{age}) \times \text{ideal weight in kg}}{85 \times \text{serum creatinine (mg/dL)}}$

Extended Interval Gentamicin/Tobramycin Therapy	
GFR (mL/min)	**Gentamicin/Tobramycin Dosage Frequency**
>60	7 mg/kg every 24 hours
40-59	7 mg/kg every 36 hours
20-39	7 mg/kg every 48 hours
<20	Extended interval not recommended

Each dose is administer over 60 minutes. Therapeutic range is a peak level of 20-30 mcg/mL and a trough level of <1.0 mcg/mL (during the 4 hours before the next dose). Monitor renal function and hearing status.

Commonly Used Abbreviations

½ NS	0.45% saline solution		tomography
ac	ante cibum (before meals)	CVP	central venous pressure
		CXR	Chest X-ray
ABG	arterial blood gas	d/c	discharge; discontinue
ac	before meals	D5W	5% dextrose water solution; also D10W, D50W
ACTH	adrenocorticotropic hormone		
ad lib	ad libitum (desired)	DIC	disseminated intravascular coagulation
ADH	antidiuretic hormone		
AFB	acid-fast bacillus	diff	differential count
alk phos	alkaline phosphatase	DKA	diabetic ketoacidosis
ALT	alanine amino-transferase	dL	deciliter
		DOSS	docusate sodium sulfo-succinate
am	morning		
AMA	against medical advice	DTs	delirium tremens
amp	ampule	ECG	electrocardiogram
AMV	assisted mandatory ventilation; assist mode ventilation	ER	emergency room
		ERCP	endoscopic retrograde cholangiopancreatography
ANA	antinuclear antibody	ESR	erythrocyte sedimentation rate
ante	before		
AP	anteroposterior	ET	endotracheal tube
ARDS	adult respiratory distress syndrome	ETOH	alcohol
		FEV_1	forced expiratory volume (in one second)
ASA	acetylsalicylic acid		
AST	aspartate amino-transferase	FiO2	fractional inspired oxygen
		g	gram(s)
bid	bis in die (twice a day)	GC	gonococcal; gonococcus
B-12	vitamin B-12 (cyanocobalamin)	GFR	glomerular filtration rate
		GI	gastrointestinal
BM	bowel movement	gm	gram
BP	blood pressure	gt	drop
BUN	blood urea nitrogen	gtt	drops
c/o	complaint of	h	hour
c	cum (with)	H_2O	water
C and S	culture and sensitivity	HBsAG	hepatitis B surface antigen
C	centigrade	HCO_3	bicarbonate
Ca	calcium	Hct	hematocrit
cap	capsule	HDL	high-density lipoprotein
CBC	complete blood count; includes hemoglobin, hematocrit, red blood cell indices, white blood cell count, and platelets	Hg	mercury
		Hgb	hemoglobin concentration
		HIV	human immunodeficiency virus
		hr	hour
cc	cubic centimeter	hs	hora somni (bedtime, hour of sleep)
CCU	coronary care unit		
cm	centimeter	IM	intramuscular
CMF	cyclophosphamide, methotrexate, fluorouracil	I and O	intake and output--measurement of the patient's intake and output
CNS	central nervous system	IU	international units
CO_2	carbon dioxide	ICU	intensive care unit
COPD	chronic obstructive pulmonary disease	IgM	immunoglobulin M
		IMV	intermittent mandatory ventilation
CPK-MB	myocardial-specific CPK isoenzyme	INH	isoniazid
		INR	International normalized ratio
CPR	cardiopulmonary resuscitation		
		IPPB	intermittent positive-pressure breathing
CSF	cerebrospinal fluid		
CT	computerized	IV	intravenous or

	intravenously	pAO₂	partial pressure of oxygen in alveolar gas
IVP	intravenous pyelogram; intravenous piggyback	PB	phenobarbital
K⁺	potassium	pc	after meals
kcal	kilocalorie	pCO2	partial pressure of carbon dioxide
KCL	potassium chloride		
KPO₄	potassium phosphate	PEEP	positive end-expiratory pressure
KUB	x-ray of abdomen (kidneys, ureters, bowels)	per	by
L	liter	pH	hydrogen ion concentration (H+)
LDH	lactate dehydrogenase	PID	pelvic inflammatory disease
LDL	low-density lipoprotein	pm	afternoon
liq	liquid	PO	orally, per os
LLQ	left lower quadrant	pO₂	partial pressure of oxygen
LP	lumbar puncture, low potency	polys	polymorphonuclear leukocytes
LR	lactated Ringer's (solution)	PPD	purified protein derivative
MB	myocardial band	PR	per rectum
MBC	minimal bacterial concentration	prn	pro re nata (as needed)
mcg	microgram	PT	physical therapy; pro-thrombin time
mEq	milliequivalent		
mg	milligram	PTCA	percutaneous transluminal coronary angioplasty
Mg	magnesium		
MgSO₄	Magnesium Sulfate	PTT	partial thromboplastin time
MI	myocardial infarction	PVC	premature ventricular contraction
MIC	minimum inhibitory concentration	q	quaque (every) q6h, q2h every 6 hours; every 2 hours
mL	milliliter		
mm	millimeter	qid	quarter in die (four times a day)
MOM	Milk of Magnesia		
MRI	magnetic resonance imaging	qAM	every morning
Na	sodium	qd	quaque die (every day)
NaHCO₃	sodium bicarbonate	qh	every hour
Neuro	neurologic	qhs	every night before bedtime
NG	nasogastric		
NKA	no known allergies	qid	4 times a day
NPH	neutral protamine Hagedorn (insulin)	qOD	every other day
NPO	nulla per os (nothing by mouth)	qs	quantity sufficient
		R/O	rule out
NS	normal saline solution (0.9%)	RA	rheumatoid arthritis; room air; right atrial
NSAID	nonsteroidal anti-inflammatory drug	Resp	respiratory rate
		RL	Ringer's lactated solution (also LR)
O₂	oxygen	ROM	range of motion
OD	right eye	rt	right
oint	ointment	s	sine (without)
OS	left eye	s/p	status post
Osm	osmolality	sat	saturated
OT	occupational therapy	SBP	systolic blood pressure
OTC	over the counter	SC	subcutaneously
OU	each eye	SIADH	syndrome of inappropriate antidiuretic hormone
oz	ounce	SL	sublingually under tongue
p, post	after	SLE	systemic lupus erythematosus
pc	post cibum (after meals)		
PA	posteroanterior; pulmonary artery	SMA-12	sequential multiple analysis; a panel of 12 chemistry tests. Tests include Na⁺, K⁺, HCO3 , chloride, BUN, glucose,
PaO₂	arterial oxygen pressure		

	creatinine, bilirubin, calcium, total protein, albumin, alkaline phosphatase.
SMX	sulfamethoxazole
sob	shortness of breath
sol	solution
SQ	under the skin
ss	one-half
STAT	statim (immediately)
susp	suspension
tid	ter in die (three times a day)
T4	Thyroxine level (T4)
tab	tablet
TB	tuberculosis
Tbsp	tablespoon
Temp	temperature
TIA	transient ischemic attack
tid	three times a day
TKO	to keep open, an infusion rate (500 mL/24h)
TMP-SMX	trimethoprim-sulfamethoxazole combination
TPA	tissue plasminogen activator
TSH	thyroid-stimulating hormone
tsp	teaspoon
U	units
UA	urinalysis
URI	upper respiratory infection
Ut Dict	as directed
UTI	urinary tract infection
VAC	vincristine, adriamycin, and cyclophosphamide
vag	vaginal
VC	vital capacity
VDRL	Venereal Disease Research Laboratory
VF	ventricular function
V fib	ventricular fibrillation
VLDL	very low-density lipoprotein
Vol	volume
VS	vital signs
VT	ventricular tachycardia
W	water
WBC	white blood count
x	times

Index